SURVIVAL

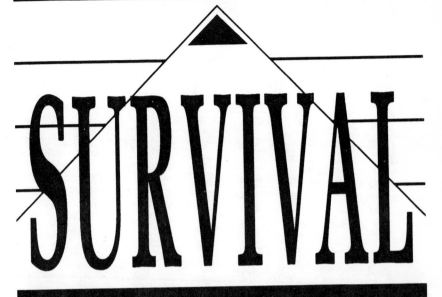

SURVIVAL

A Manual That Could Save Your Life

Chris & Gretchen Janowsky

PALADIN PRESS
BOULDER, COLORADO

Survival: A Manual That Could Save Your Life
by Chris and Gretchen Janowsky

Copyright © 1986 by Chris and Gretchen Janowsky

Paladin Press 1989 edition published with permission
from Graphic North Printing.

ISBN 0-87364-506-5
Printed in the United States of America

Published by Paladin Press, a division of
Paladin Enterprises, Inc., P.O. Box 1307,
Boulder, Colorado 80306, USA.
(303) 443-7250

Direct inquiries and/or orders to the above address.

DEDICATION

I'd like to dedicate this book to my children, Liana, Lance and Jesse; and to what's left of mankind. If by chance it saves one life it was all worth it.

TABLE OF CONTENTS

FOREWORD

Let me begin with a little on how, where and why this book was written. Each page, in one way or another, is in actuality a part of my life and the information herein has not only been tested but lived so many times that it is not only a workable system for wilderness survival, but has become an enjoyable, rewarding way of life. Each word had been written by the light of the long arctic summer days with its beautiful midnight sun, or by the light of my kerosene lamp during the long winter evenings and days of darkness and shadows. The birds watch me write through the cabin window from the planter where I feed them.

The lynx sneaks by; he thinks I don't see him. And my friend the snow white Ermine is everywhere. There is a small Boreal owl who sings to me each winter evening, and the red squirrels who are in everything but still are my friends. My two hard-working, trusting dogs lie on the floor near the wood stove. They must wonder why I spend so much time with a pen and paper. I've also been blessed with the good fortune to have the companionship and help of a wonderful wife. My cabin is a happy cabin, filled with peace and it's good. These, along with the love of my children, are my most priceless treasures. I couldn't possibly want any more than this life of peace and harmony.

The purpose of this book is many-fold. First is to teach anyone who would like to learn true wilderness survival skills in a proven, practical, unforgetable way; to teach some of the secrets to things we have given away in trade for a modern plastic lifestyle, and to help develop a positive way of thinking which is the answer to so many questions in life. People are constantly asking us "Don't you ever get cabin fever?" To be honest, I really don't know what cabin fever is. All I know is I haven't had time to get it because Gretchen and I have been to busy being happy and for us there's not enough time in the day to enjoy all that has been given us and to learn the secrets that are all around us.

Survival to me is life, so L.I.F.E. has become the name of this book and L.I.F.E. is the acronym of the system. Remember the word life, it's your key to being rescued or walking out, and the system is your secret potion to change what could be an ordeal or tragedy into an organized system of living, enjoying it, and becoming one with nature instead of fighting it. To fight it is to lose; to respect it, to learn from it, and become in harmony with it is to win.

A good example of this attitude is when I came face to face with one of the biggest grizzlies I have ever seen. A full-grown grizzly bear is the largest land carnivore in North America. He's fast enough to catch a horse and strong enough to kill anything he catches. A grizzly bear can break the neck of a 900 pound moose with one swat and I was in his way. What did I do? I could have stood my ground and stayed on the trail that was rightfully his, and confronted a 700 pound killing machine, equipped with a mouth full of 2¼" razor blades and paws as big as my head with five each rather impressive looking 4" claws. I could have run but surely he would have caught me. In my opinion trying to be a hero and stupidity are one and the same. I got off the bear's path and out of his way. He continued on his way and seemingly never gave me a second thought. He obviously didn't think of me as much of a threat.

1

The interesting thing I learned (right after I regained some composure) was that he allowed me room in his world as long as I wasn't trying to change it. I've walked the same path several times after and have seen him only one more time. This time I was hunting and a good distance from him. I allowed him to pass and for the first time I knew how the bear felt when we first met. And I'd swear his eyes spoke to me and said you've learned well, my friend and now we must each go our own way in peace. I've never seen him since; I'll never forget the look in his eyes. I'll always respect him, as he did me, and remember what he taught me, and the warning I'll never forget.

My wife and I teach wilderness and medical survival in Alaska, our home, and travel most anywhere in the lower 48 and Canada to teach groups of men, women and children. In this day and age more then ever I believe there is a very serious need for this training everywhere. Each year so many people die needlessly because of hysteria, ignorance, or over confidence of their own abilities. There is book after book written on survival using 150 pounds of unneeded gear that you would need a pack horse or sled dog team to haul, but when the unexpected happens you don't have it with you. And just as bad is the kit that claims "everything you need" and at the same time fits in your shirt pocket. It's really hard to cut fire wood with a razor blade and a plastic tube tent, when it's really cold, makes an inexpensive coffin.

In this book I will try to teach you all I can but there is no substitute for actual training. Read what I have to say and practice what you learn. In your backyard, in your house, anywhere, but practice what you learn, **now**, not when you need it most. The practice experience can be fun and can become a family activity. Our children have a great time building snow caves and shelters in the winter. And they don't even know they are learning. They think it's funny to be able to start a fire with flint and steel faster than a grown up with matches. Make a game with your whole family out of what you learn here and live to play another game. It's the most valuable life insurance you've ever invested in.

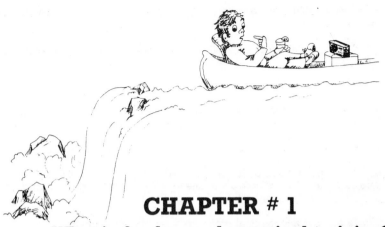

CHAPTER # 1

What is & who needs survival training?

Of course everyone knows how to survive in this world, and you would never end up in a really serious situation. For sure it will always happen to someone else. Or you don't need it, you had a few hours of it 20 years ago in the military—of course you can't recall very much of it but you're all set.

It's for these reasons hundreds of people die each year. It just wasn't going to happen to them. Through our search and rescue bush medical work we find this misconception the # 1 killer. Anyone that operates a snow machine, flies in airplanes, drives a car, or lives, needs to know how to survive on their own. What would you do right now if the snow was coming down so fast you couldn't even see 3 feet in front of you. And now after the extremely heavy snow load the power goes out. You have lost all light and heat for an indefinite period of time. The roads are now impassable and it's even snowing harder. The temperature has dropped drastically in the last two days and you find even your water service is frozen. That's never going to happen to you of course, but that's what the people of the Buffalo area said before the killing blizzard of '77, and again, so many people never expected it to happen to them. People caught on the roads died in their cars and other died trying to walk to safety. It was a needless waste of human life.

The folllowing is a test we give at the beginning of our classes. Take out a pencil and see how many questions you can answer correctly before reading any further. If you can answer them all your chances of surviving a serious survival situation right now is excellent. If you score 80% your chances are good; if you score less than 70% you could very well become a statistic.

1.) You are in a wilderness survival situation and it is 40° below, you have to shelter-in, make camp for over night, ect. Approximately how much water do you have to drink to avoid dehydration?

2.) You are out in the cold, −40°, and you realize that one of your feet is actually frozen and you are five miles from your cabin or help. What should you do for your foot?

3.) When reaching shelter what is the specific therapy for a deep frozen extremity?

4.) Most hypothermia deaths occur in the _____ to _____ temperature range.

5.) When performing one-rescuer cardiopulmonary resuscitation, chest compressions should be at the rate of _____ per minute.

6.) Anaphylactic shock is caused by _____ .

7.) As you should know, water hemlock is poisonous. How can you positively identify it from other similar looking edible plants such as cow parsnip?

8.) What is the normal loop size of a snare intended for snowshoe hare?

9.) The magnetic force of the earth pulls the compass needle out of line with true north and this is called declination. This declination can very up to _____ degrees in the U.S..

10.) Is alcohol a beneficial warming agent when a person is becoming hypothermic?

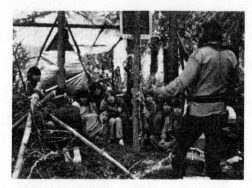

ANSWERS

1.) Up to 8 quarts in 12 hours.

2.) Nothing. Do not thaw the foot until you have reached secure shelter where there is no danger of re-freezing the foot.

3.) Rapid thaw in water approximately 110°F.

4.) 30° to 50° above zero F.

5.) 80

6.) Severe allergic reactions, such as to insect stings.

7.) Hemlock has chambers in the root stalk.

8.) Approximately 4" diameter.

9.) 30

10.) No

The test you just took was not designed to be hard but to touch on a wide range of extremely important skills that everyone should know in daily life and some are especially important in a wilderness survival situation. For instance, questions # 1-6 are strictly medical and every man and woman should know the answers. If you didn't, right now is the time to learn. It could mean your life or the life of someone you care about.

Question # 7 naturally relates to edible and poisonous wild plants. To some readers this may not seem applicable to them but in a wilderness survival situation it could mean life or death.

Question # 8 is again in the area of wild food procurement, this time in the form of meat which gives life sustaining protein and minerals, a slow-release energy source, and a damaged tissue rebuilder.

Question # 9 relates to direction finding and it's surprising how many people have compasses and really don't understand them. Most people feel when a compass reads north, north is in that direction. As you can see, that is a very serious misconception, and could get you very lost and extremely dead.

Question # 10 deals solely with the treatment of an already hypothermic person. This area of your medical knowledge can't be stressed too much, considering that it is one of the three major killers of human beings that end up in a survival situation.

My objective here is not to frighten you but to make you aware of how so many men, women and children die each year in unforseen survival situations. And it can happen to you without you planning it. It's how you react and what you do about the situation that will determine whether you live or die. Your life now is in your hands.

Your plan now is L.I.F.E., what this book is about. This book is L.I.F.E., the way to survive. L.I.F.E. is the comprehensive survival system that keeps you mentally and physically strong and healthy—and a survivor. The L.I.F.E. system has 4 steps you must take in proper sequence and you will live through a survival ordeal.

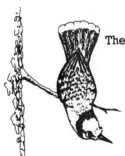

The 4 steps of L.I.F.E. are:

L - Logically gather your thoughts and composure and assess the situation.
I - Inventory the materials, tools, and equipment available.
F - Formulate a plan.
E - Enact your plan in a positive manner.

Let me here introduce my friend, Flapjack, a grey jay who chose to spend time with me. Just as he taught me some things about his world, let him guide you through the lessons of this book.

L.I.F.E. - Logic, Inventory, Formulation, and Enactment.

Now it's time to look at and understand the "L.I.F.E. system". Learn the tricks and how to apply them to any situation. Gather and store the knowledge that will make you a survivor, just as the small red squirrel does with the spruce seeds to insure his survival through the cold winter. The knowledge you gain and store is the seeds that will get you through what could be for most people a tragedy.

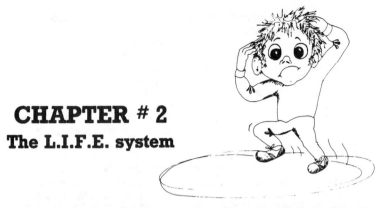

CHAPTER # 2
The L.I.F.E. system

Logic - attitude and situation assessment

To begin, logic and attitude go hand and hand. If your attitude is poor and negative, your mind will not be allowed to think logically. And if you allow this situation to take control, your problems will inevitably be compounded. If you are in a serious situation the last thing you need is more problems. You have already had more than your share of problems created for you. You don't need to create more for yourself.

You must have a **POSITIVE** outlook on the entire situation. There's nothing you can do to change what has already happened. Whether it was your fault or not doesn't matter any more. It has happened, and what you do from now on will save your life and possibly the lives of others.

First of all you have the most positive thing in the whole world going for you right away. You're alive. So instead of feeling bad for yourself, feel good because you are alive. Your only problem now is staying that way, and it starts with this attitude. I heard a little satirical jingle once when I was a young boy and I've repeated it many times since when I've been in danger or confused. It went, "When in danger or in doubt, run in circles, scream and shout". It makes me laugh, settle down, and compose myself. It reminds me how stupid panic makes a person and how useless he or she becomes. Let's face it, if you run in circles at best all you can get is tired, and you can scream and shout your lungs out in the wilderness but there is no one to hear.

It would be my advice to take a more positive logical approach to the situation. So if you end up in a serious survival situation and things look really bad, it might not hurt to repeat that little satire—it sure makes me feel better. This is an important milestone in survival. Your attitude is now positive and you're alive. I also find at this time it helps to sit down for a while and say a prayer. This has always helped me, and when things are really bad I can use all the help I can get. Again a positive attitude is being built and strengthened. Now and only now can I look at the situation logically and make the proper situation assessment.

Your situation assessment is the next most important thing you can do. Your future depends on it so it must be right. What exactly is a situation assessment? It is looking at all the positive and negative aspects of your particular situation. Your two main concerns at this point will always be shelter and water, unless you are sure you can easily walk out and you know exactly where you are going. If the latter is not the case, you will be sheltering-in for the night and tomorrow you will have a better capacity to make that deci-

7

sion. Now it is time to look around you and notice everything that might be to your advantage and disadvantage. Once you've done this you must weigh things out and start making logical decisions.

If you are in an area with an abundance of fuel for a fire this would be a positive reason to stay put. Fire is not only an important tool, and a source of heat, but also a great psychological uplift. We will cover this in the chapter on fire but for now it's a positive reason for staying. Second, if there is an abundance of fuel for fire there probably is an abundance of easy shelter building material. This certainly is another logical reason for staying. If it's winter and there is snow on the ground your water supply problem is over, another plus.

The winter with its cold also brings snow, and snow more than not, is your friend. In this hypothetical case where most people might consider winter a liability, things are actually looking pretty good. And remember those first two main concerns, shelter and water, are taken care of. And it's lack of shelter and water that bring on the two main killers in the wild, hypothermia and dehydration, and not necessarily in that order. (We will be covering these two serious conditions later.)

It's at this point where many people make a very serious mistake. It's getting dark or is probably already dark, and they decide out of panic to start walking, or I should say stumbling, around in the woods. Under no circumstances should anyone try to walk through a forest at night. If you think you have problems now, think what it would be like in that forest if you were blind from poking your eyes out on branches. Or you fell and broke a leg. At night stay put, enjoy the fire, get some rest and drink as much water as you possibly can. Tomorrow will come soon enough and if you wake up early you may start your day with a beautiful sunrise, something most people don't take the time to enjoy anymore. And just because you are lost doesn't mean you can't start to appreciate and enjoy the beautiful things around you.

If you happen to be in a northern spruce forest your first early morning visit will probably be from a gray jay, commonly called a camp robber or whisky jack. He is a great opportunist and many lessons can be learned from him. Besides that now you have someone to talk to. If you by chance have any food at all with you don't leave it where he might find it or it's as good as gone. Don't frighten him away—in the future you may have to have him for dinner. This may sound cruel but you too have to become an opportunist, just like the jay.

Everything you see from now on is part of your situation assessment. Now that you've seen a beautiful sunrise and made a new friend, it's time to look around and evaluate your surroundings. Are you in a good place to be seen and rescued? These and many more are the questions you must ask yourself and then come up with an intelligent, logical answer. This is your situation assessment and it's very important. Your life depends on it and L.I.F.E. is what this is all about.

At this point you have already engaged the L.I.F.E. system in your situation. And now let's take a look back at what you've done so far. You've initiated "L" which was to logically gather your thoughts and assess your situation. You've seen a beautiful sunrise, you've made a new friend, you've in a good logical frame of mind and you're alive. A little hungry maybe, but very much alive.

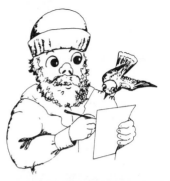

Now that you've survived your first night in the wilderness and you've made the first part of L.I.F.E. work for you, it's time to initiate the second step: "I"—inventory. You must inventory the materials you have at hand. You must look very closely at everything you have on you and around you. Nothing should be overlooked. If it was an aircraft you went down in, you're already set. The aircraft will make a poor cold weather shelter but most everything you need to survive is there. The oil in the crank case will burn and so will the gasoline. There may (and should) be a survival kit on board, maybe even a rifle and ammunition. The foam rubber in the seats makes excellent fire-starter, or warm foot protection. The glass makes a good signaling device. The aircraft itself, if down in the right place, may make a perfect signal just by being there. The cables that control the aircraft make fine snares, and maybe the radio is still working. If the aircraft has a battery in it you can make sparks to make your fire. You may have a knife in your pocket, and maybe a plastic sandwich bag. Even though by now you would rather have the sandwich that came in it, don't throw it out. If there are tires on the aircraft they will make a thick black smoke when thrown in a signal fire (let the air out first).

These are just some examples of your inventory, and the list goes on and on. What's very important is that no matter what it is, you can probably use it in one way or another. Just as important is the inventory of the natural resources around you. This is another area where most people fail. The spruce tree for example, is probably the best friend a man or animal in the north ever had. You can burn its wood to make heat to keep you warm, dry your clothers, and make water from snow. The cambium layer of the tree is rich in nutrients including vitamin C. The pitch is edible and rich in vitamin C, also an excellent wound closure like sutures. The young needles are edible and the whole beautiful tree is shelter building material to keep you warm, dry and alive.

What else might you find and inventory from nature's store house? Snow is a good item. It can make you a fine shelter even at 80° below zero and affords you life-sustaining water. It helps you in tracking and setting up your trap line, it can also help you in signaling for help. An abundance of animal tracks means food, and soon needed protein. A frozen lake or river may mean fish.

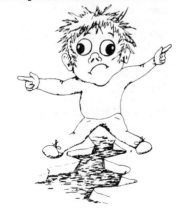

These are a few examples of your inventory and more will be covered in the following chapters. This is an important part of your survival and the L.I.F.E. system. This is what helps you decide whether to try to walk out or stay put. And my advice is whenever possible, to stay put, especially if someone knows you are out there.

The last two steps of the L.I.F.E. system are formulate and enact your plan.

9

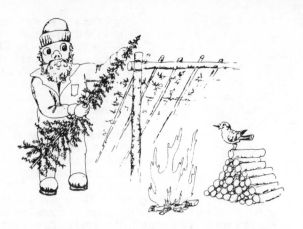

Now that you've assessed your situation and inventoried everything at hand, you know what your capabilities and goals are. You must formulate a plan to make this happen. Your first major decision here is whether or not you are going to stay where you are. If you must move to another location you should do it as quickly as possible. Time is of the essence now because if someone is looking for you, you must have your signals ready so they can spot you. Again, I must caution you on walking out—unless you have a very good reason and sense of direction, it is usually a poor choice. You will be burning a tremendous number of calories, you will be subject to the elements, you may not be able to set up a permanent, effective signaling procedure, and you probably will literally walk yourself to death.

But whatever your plan may be, now is the time to enact it. Two simple examples of this would be: number one, you have decided to walk out. Your plan must include what direction you will travel, a way of keeping on that course and a time schedule of how long you plan to walk each day. You must allow enough time to set up overnight camp and have some way of signaling should an airplane fly over. There again, are many more considerations that must be part of your walking out decision, but this is a good example of how to formulate your plan.

In the second case you have decided to stay put. Your plan now must include immediately, setting up your signal system. The search plane, or any aircraft, could be in sight any minute and you must be ready at that time. Next, you must decide the location and style of your permanent camp. This must be near your signals. You must consider your water source and what you are going to eat. These are just a few parts of your entire plan. The order of your plan is very important and signaling now will be # 1.

If this was a real survival situation and you had followed the L.I.F.E. system this far, you would be in control and in pretty good shape. Remember, you are alive and intend to stay that way. The only thing you need now is the knowledge of a multitude of wilderness and medical survival skills. The following chapters contain these skills, tricks and techniques, and **NOW** is the time to learn them, not when you need them most.

CHAPTER # 3
The Survival Kit

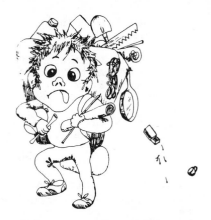

The survival kit and what it contains depends on your knowledge, adaptability to any situation, and practicality. For the most part, what is in a survival kit is relative to your knowledge. Simply, the more you know the less equipment you will need to achieve the same goal. In most cases the survival kit should contain everything you **NEED** but be limited in size and weight. All survival equipment in your kit should be of first-class material. This is no place to cheat on quality and you should think of your kit as your life line. I will be listing my own two personal sets of kits. Sets meaning 1 survival kit, and 1 first aid kit. Set # 1 is the small belt model which is with me always. Set # 2 is larger and goes with me whenever I travel in a car, truck, horseback, snow machine, airplane, etc. When I get back home it is always hung by the door.

Because I teach survival I've had so many calls for these kits I now make them for my students, readers, or any one else that would like them. I am sure many readers would like to make up their own and save a little money although it doesn't usually work out that way. The choice is yours and the important thing is that you end up with the kits exactly like I have designed them. There should be no deviation from quantity or quality. Each item has one or more important use. Each item has been field tested over and over again and has been found extremely useful, if not essential. Kit # 1-a. Survival Belt Kit consists of: 1 - **belt pack** approx. 4" wide X 5" high X 2" deep - set up with individual compartments and constructed from nylon pack cloth; 1 - small folding knife of good quality with a blade of approx. 3"; 1 - knife sharpener; 1 - flint at least 2" long; 1 - large saftey pin; 1 - tape (water proof); 1 - ziplock plastic bag; 1 - nylon twine; 1 - wire ring saw; 1 - container of fire starter; 1 - flashlight—micro lith; 1 - spool of wire; 1 - gaff hook; 1 - nail; 3 - small animal snares; 1 - fishing kit with assorted hooks, dry flies, split shot, jigs, leader, line, metal lures and plastic baits; 1 - metal signal mirror.

In a survival situation this kit is a necessity and will get you by nicely if you know all the ways to use its contents. And remember it is only 4" X 5" X 2", not too bulky to have with you always. A survival kit is of no use if it's not with you when you need it. Let us now take a closer look at this small kit. The small folding knife must be of good quality with one or two blades. It must hold an edge well and sharpen easily. One of the two blades should be at least 3" long. This knife will be a major tool for your survival. It will be used for everything from shaving small pieces of wood for fire starter, cleaning fish and game, to striking the flint to make your fire. It is essential that it is a good knife.

In my tests I have learned that "E-Z Lap" diamond knife sharpener is the finest and safest sharpener of its size. It's expensive but I've found through repeated use, cut fingers can result from many of the more inexpensive types. This you can not afford in the field. Also it comes in two pieces, the handle section can be used as a straw to siphon surface water from areas where it would be next to impossible to collect it. Also because of the sharpener's style it can become a perfect marlin spike (used for untying knots).

Your flint will take the place of all matches. A flint and steel (in this case your folding knife) will start hundreds of fires, and as quickly as matches. And another distinct advantage is that they aren't affected by water or dampness. Along with this is your container of home-made fire starter which you'll find is truely an amazingly quick way to start a fire. There is enough of the fire starter material in the container to start at least 40 fires, and long before that time you will have accumulated some of nature's fire starter.

The plastic bag is to be used for water collection only and should be well taken care of, although if you do puncture it, there is waterproof repair tape wrapped around the E-Z Lap sharpener handle. There is 21 ft. of 42 lb. nylon twine that will hang your water generator, help make your shelter, and perform a multitude of other functions.

The small ring saw works well on small jobs like shelter building. A larger saw would make things somewhat easier but the size would defeat the compactness of the belt kit.

The micro-lith flashlight is the only way to go; it's compact, bright, and its battery has an extremely long shelf life. It, like so many other items, has more than one use. It's magnifying lense will start a fire with the aid of the sun and the main body of light can be used for a water collecter.

The 3 snares are intended, naturally, for food procurement and the spool of wire is for making more snares if needed, shelter building, and probably at least another 100 uses.

The gaff hook is intended to aid you in fishing but as you will find, has other uses. The small complete fishing kit will supply you with fish if they are available, and the signal mirror, if used properly can give your location to a search party.

As you can see, the small kit contains the important tools needed to help perform the necessary functions of wilderness survival: water procurement, shelter, fire starter, food procurement, and signaling help.

There are many other items that can compliment this small kit and that's where the larger kit comes in. But remember, with the proper knowledge you can "get by" with these few essential tools.

We also build custom survival parkas, which are survival and medical kits themselves. So each time you put the parka on you have with you for that unplanned emergency, the equipment to save your life. It's a good compliment to the small kits and in a survival situation will make a person even more comfortable and make the work easier.

Whenever I am traveling, hunting, camping, or fishing, a large kit goes with me and with that kit I can stay in the wilderness permanently in a comfortable manner.

And just as important as the survival kits, are the medical kits. The small medical kit that is worn on the belt with the survival kit contains: 1 - sterile 2" Kling bandage; 1 - tweezers; 1 - scissors; 5 - bandaids; 1 - package of tums; 4 - sterile 3" X 3" dressings; 4 - sterile 4" X 4" dressings; 1 - sterile adaptic 4" X 4" dressing; 1 - 3½" X 5" moleskin; 4 - individual application tubes triple antibiotic ointment; 1 - eyewash applicator full of saline solution; 1 - package of aspirin; 1 - triangular bandage; 4 - alcohol prep pads;

4 - butterfly bandages. This kit will get you by in most instances and could very well save your life.

The following is the list of items in the large survival kit. The kit is break-away so that the medical section can be seperated from the survival section. Both sections are the same size and are fitted with shoulder pack straps so they can be worn by two different people or put together to make one complete survival and medical kit. Sewing awl; needle nose pliers with wire cutter; needle; dental floss (for sewing); folding knife; Seirra saw (folding); ring saw; survival saw; snow shovel; visqueen; water generator; signal cloth (3' X 3'); fishing equipment: 3 large safety pins, 18 lb. test nylon line—50 yds., leader, misc. hooks of varied sizes, various flies, lures, jigs and plastic bait, gaff hook, split shot, fish spear and fly dope; multiple vitamins; protein tablets; hard candy; dried eggs; dried milk; tent cloth; file; silverware; 3 space blankets; compass; signal mirror; 2 sky blazers; 4 candles; micro-lith flashlight; extra battery; extra bulb; fire starter; matches (wind proof/water proof); butane lighter; flint; bug dope (GI); 12 snares; spool snare wire; plastic drinking tube; 2 heavy zip lock bags; p-38 can opener; water purification tablets; sling shot rubber and ammunition; diamond knife sharpener; whistle; towel and face cloth; soap; 2 orange smoke signals; 75 yds. 42 lb. nylon twine; 75 ft. nylon cord; 1 pair work gloves; metal cup; mess kit; small grill; mouse trap; 1 roll surveyors tape and folding water jug.

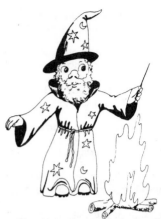

CHAPTER # 4
Wilderness Skill # 1
The Magic Fire

Fire in most survival situations has no substitute for its psychological up lift and the tranquilizing effect it lends to the human brain. As you know, when you are acting with a calm and tranquil state of mind you conserve energy; your decision making process becomes more active and accurate, fewer accidents happen and you become a generally happy person. I find that fire always helps in the endeavor. Think back on how many times you've stared into the flames of a fireplace or campfire, sometimes perhaps for hours. You do it because it makes you feel good.

People that go camping together nearly every night find themselves enevitably sitting around the campfire. When each new group of students show up at my training camp we spend that first special evening getting aquainted around the campfire. The fire is magic and you'll find that it is a work-saving tool that is there for you to use. Fire is beneficial physically, naturally, because it will help keep you warm, makes many foods palatable, can change certain poisonous plants into life-saving edible delights, will run a water generator for you, purify drinking water, dry your clothes, and be a signal for either day or night rescue.

As I sit in my cabin right now and look out at the 40° below environment around it, I know that the fire in my stove makes it all so easy. At the same time, to take full advantage of that life giving heat, there is a pot of moose stew simmering and giving the air a wonderful aroma. Yes, fire is a magic gift to mankind. So let's study the important skill of fire making.

I've had the good fortune to have spent some time with an extremely woods-wise Indian who was also a trapper. He told me that when it came to fire the big difference between most white men and most Indians is that the white man builds a big fire and sits back a long ways from it, and the Indian builds a small fire and sits real close. This makes a lot of sense and shouldn't be forgotten. A small fire consumes less fuel and your body burns less valuable energy gathering the fuel. Always remember during a wilderness survival situation, energy conservation is of # 1 concern.

Fire Making Materials

One of your first decisions upon making camp is whether or not you are going to have a fire. If the answer is yes, is there a ample supply of fuel near by? If so, next you must have a means of igniting the fuel. There are several ways this can be accomplished and the list below will explain them. I have tested almost every way known to start a fire in the wilderness and have found nothing as good, as fast, and as reliable as flint and steel.

Flint and Steel Occupies little space, always works under all weather conditions. Just 2″ of flint is good for hundreds of lights. This is the method taught at my school and it never fails.

Matches Work very well under ideal conditions, will not work if wet, are not reusable and take up too much room per amounts of lights. Highly affected by wind, not affected by cold.

Water Proof Matches Work very well under most conditions including dampness. They are not reusable, take up too much room, highly affected by wind, not affected by cold.

Water Proof - Wind Proof Matches A superior match. Work well under most conditions including dampness and wind. Take up too much room. Not affected by cold. They also need a dry striking surface.

Electric Spark Any vehicle which has a wet cell battery is a ignition source. Contact of the wires with a scraping motion will create sparks.

Flares Will start a fire almost anywhere but shouldn't be wasted if there is another way.

Magnifying Glass All convex lenses can be used in bright sun light conditions to concentrate the sun's rays to one singular point of intense heat. Needs an intense light source.

Friction There are many methods under this section but they all require practice. The bow and drill is probably one of the easiest of this group. I teach this skill at my school but it requires energy so I don't advise it if there are easier methods available.

Now that you have a way of making a spark or flame, you will need something to light. The next material we will call fire starter and is something more flameable than tinder, which will be your next item, then kindling, and finally your fuel supply, usually larger pieces of wood.

In my survival kit I have a flint and the knife is the steel. I also have a water proof match container that is filled with cotton batten soaked with vaseline. A small piece of the cotton and a spark from the flint, and presto, I have a fire every time. The fire starter burns long enough and hot enough to get almost any tinder or small kindling going. The method will work under windy, wet or extremely cold conditions. The nice part is that there can be over 100 lights from the small match container of fire starter and the flint will hardly be used. I use my pre-made fire starter if necessary, and whenever possible use the natural fire starters I find in the bush. This gives me a back up, fool-proof system that is on my hip, still ready for use in case of a more severe survival situation, such as a medical accident where I can't move far and need instant heat.

There are many sources of tinder or fire starter available to you. Like I mentioned earlier, cotton batten soaked in vaseline is excellent. The cotton alone works well, but when soaked in vaseline, burns hotter and longer. Cotton bandages in your first aid kit will double as fire starter, as will cotton threads and lint from your clothes, shredded string, and rope, powdered wood, small fine pieces of birch bark, spruce and pine pitch.

Just remember all tinder must be bone-dry. Tinder can be made to burn more easily by adding gunpowder from a cartridge, a squirt of most liquid insect repellents (the military type is extremely flamable); a few drops of gasoline, if available; alcohol prep pads from your first aid kit; fuzzy material scraped from plants; the black moss hanging on the dead squaw wood branches of spruce trees; birds' nests and field mouse nests. When you find good tinder and fire starter, save some and dry it in the sun or by the fire so you will have it for the next fire. Paraffin from a candle also helps start a fire.

Now that we have ignited a small fire we must have some sort of kindling within arm's reach to add to it. It can be small slivers of dry wood that you made with your knife, small squaw wood, feather sticks, etc. This is the material that will get your fire going so larger fuel can be added. You must have a substantial amount of this kindling nearby to insure a proper base for the fuel that you will be adding on top. Remember, no matter what you add to your fire, be careful not to smother it. Fire needs oxygen to burn and it must come to the fire from underneath.

Once you are at the point of adding fuel, the skills become less and the work increases. This fire you have just created wants fuel and lots of it. Standing dead wood is a good source. It burns well and can be broken over another tree. You should break it rather than cut it if you can as it takes less calories of energy. Put long pieces on the fire and let the fire do the work of burning it in two, instead of cutting it into short pieces. Once you have a substantial fire with a lot of coals you will be able to burn almost any fuel, including green wood which burns best if split. You should make some wedges out of wood to drive into the end of green wood to split it. You'll want a good supply of fuel on hand to keep your fire going and you should never hunt for it at night if at all possible. That's when accidents happen, especially to your eyes from tree branches.

Some good types of kindling you can make are feather sticks, curly cues and heart wood splinters. Even wet wood is usually dry in the center (the heart) so by splitting you will be able to get at this section. Remember to save yourself a lot of work once you have the first fire going start drying the kindling and tinder for future fires. Large pieces of fuel wood can also be dried close to the fire. Because of the environment and circumstances your fuel source may change drastically but usually there is a fuel source of some sort. Some materials you may consider as fuel are dry wood, green wood, coal, oil shale, oil sand, dry animal dung, animal fat, animal bones, dry grass braided into bunches, peat (found on undercut river banks), roots. Mosses will burn, as will drift wood if dried well.

If you are near a disabled vehicle (airplane, snow machine, etc.) you can burn gasoline, oil, or a mixture of both oil and gasoline, **with the following caution.**

Burning of Gasoline and Fuel Oil Gasoline and fuel oil can be burned safely by taking a container such as a small can and filling it with sand, dirt or fine gravel. Next fill with gasoline, but not over the sand level, add a little more sand. This now can be ignited safely. The sand acts as a catalyst for the fuel.

If it is cold and the fuel will be coming from an aircraft you just went down in, one of your first jobs will be to dump the warm engine oil into a container before it gets so cold it doesn't want to flow. The oil in that crank case will make excellent fire starter or can be a source of fuel by itself.

The foam rubber in the aircraft seats makes excellent fire starter. The foam rubber soaked in crank case oil and contained in a can will make an in-shelter heat source or small cooking stove.

One important caution to remember about your fire is that when drying clothes and equipment, do not get them too close to the fire. A burned boot or glove could prove to be a very serious mistake.

When building a single lean-to type shelter a reflector always adds to the heating efficiency. A few green logs on an incline about 12" from the far side of the fire is excellent and should always be considered when a large amount of heat is required. The reflector makes a fine cooking rack and an ideal place to stand or hang and stack future tinder and kindling for drying. I like to build the fire itself approx. 3½' from the front of the shelter, but no closer or you may have an unpleasant experience with sparks.

During snow or wet conditions, you should always build a platform underneath the fire. Stone or green wood works well. Never build your fire under a snow-laden tree or the snow may fall and extinguish your fire. I like to place large rocks or logs around the fire, not so much to contain it, but to act as a cooking platform and drying shelves. When you decide to turn in for the night, lay some larger green round logs on top-they will burn the longest, providing there is a good bed of coals. Now its time for a good night's sleep so you will have the energy for tomorrow. At this point you've accomplished a lot-you've put yourself in a good frame of mind, you're now warm and dry. You've also defeated one of your two biggest enemies-hypothermia (covered under medical).

When building your campfire, try to put the fire about 5' from standing trees or just beyond overhanging branches. This will be important for a swing pole to make water in the winter and for cooking. Your fire should always be built in a safe enough manner so as not to start a forest or grass fire. A little common sense here will go a long way. Always clear an area under and around the proposed fire location. When leaving the area for good, make sure your fire is completely out.

Important information to review.

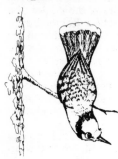

* Clear an area under and around your fire area.
* Treat gasoline with caution. **NEVER** add it to a fire or hot coals.
* Be constantly collecting fire starting materials and drying them for future use.
* Never try to dry wet clothes too close to the fire.
* Never sleep too close to your fire.
* When you break camp make sure your fire is completely out.

Some important things to know and remember about fire are:

1. Smoke rising straight up from a fire usually means fair weather. Smoke turning downward usually means stormy weather.
2. Fire can be a useful tool that will save you work and thus help you conserve valuable energy.
3. Fire or smoke from a fire is one of the finest signaling devices you could have.
4. Fire can keep you from becoming hypothermic (the # 1 cause of wilderness deaths).
5. Fire has a definite tranquilizing effect on your mind.
6. Fire makes much of your food more palatable.
7. Fire can purify water.
8. Fire can help generate water (the # 2 killer is dehydration).
9. Fire making is an important wilderness skill that should be practiced and mastered. This skill can make you a very comfortable survivor, or the lack of this skill can leave you very dead.
10. Do not attempt to burn gasoline in any way until you have learned how. Gasoline is extremely volatile and unless properly controlled will become a bomb and serious injuries or death can occur.

As Webster states, fire is the active principle of burning, characterized by heat and light of combustion, and combustion is oxidation accompanied by heat and, usually, light. What is important to remember here is the word oxidation. Oxidation is the union of a substance with oxygen. Without oxygen there will be no combustion and thus no fire. The more oxygen the fire receives the more rapid the combustion and in most cases the greater the amount of heat, and light, but a much faster burning time or life. Knowing these principles will tell you exactly what kind of fire you must build to fill your particular need and how to build it.

Considering oxygen controls the rate of combustion, understanding the hows and whys of oxygen related to fire making is extremely important. First of all, the source of oxygen is naturally, the air we breathe. The air is made up of an invisable mixture of gasses (chiefly nitrogen and oxygen, as well as hydrogen, carbon dioxide, argon, neon helium, etc.). Oxygen is the most abundant of all elements; it occurs free in the atmosphere, forming one fifth of its volume. We have and enjoy a great quantity of oxygen around us always but when used for supporting combustion it must be brought to the fuel source from underneath, (see fig. # F-1). If the flow of oxygen is increased under or at the base of the fire, combustion will be accelerated. If this amount of oxygen is reduced it will slow down the rate of combustion. In a survival situation both aspects are useful and necessary.

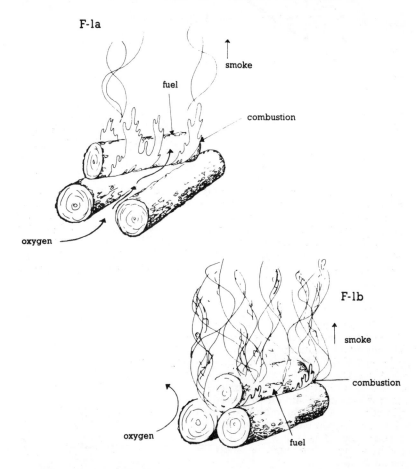

At this point it might be interesting to note that nature has supplied two of the three items needed for your fire, oxygen for combustion, and fuel. All you need supply is a source of ignition, whether it be a match or spark, and the knowledge of how to make it work.

In the next set of illustrations you will see the most common types of fires used in a wilderness survival situation.

Fig. # F-2 is the pyramid fire. The pyramid fire will burn at an extremely rapid rate, give off a tremendous amount of heat and will give off light of high intensity. The reason why this fire burns so quickly is because of all the air spaces through which oxygen can travel from below. This type of fire will make an excellent night signal fire.

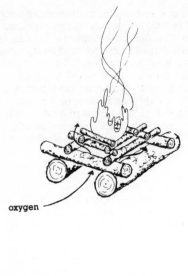

oxygen

F-3

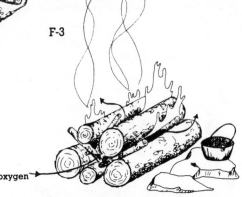

oxygen

In Fig. # F-3 your fuel, in this case logs, are laid parallel to each other in a stack. Small pieces of wood can be used to slightly separate the logs from each other, which will allow some constant oxygen flow. As the fire burns and the amount of hot coals increases, the air spaces will be made by the fire itself. This is a good fire for most general uses. It is a much slower burning fire than the pyramid fire; it gives off less heat and light but in most cases, enough to do the trick. With this type of fire you will be conserving fuel.

The Tee Pee fire illustrated in figure # F-4 is used on a small scale and to get your final fire going. If you keep building the Tee Pee larger collapse will occur. Once you have a substantial fire started in this way, slightly larger wood can be laid for whatever style of fire you choose to build over it. It will be a good base for a pyramid or stack fire. It is a low heat and moderate light fire with a short untended life.

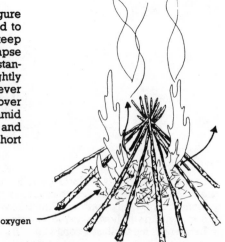

oxygen

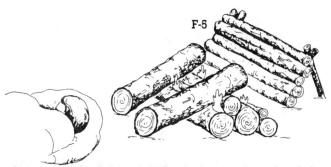

F-5

I've always used the safety night fire in the evening when I sleep in the wilderness. It enables me to stay closer to the fire without the fear of a log from my night stack fire, rolling onto me. The two slanted logs should be green and of substantial weight to keep a pressure against the fire. As the fire burns and settles it will be pushed away from me, my shelter, and my gear. This is illustrated in figure # F-5. The fire itself will have a good base of hot coals, a layer of dry round wood, with the remainder upper level of green wood. Leaving as few air spaces as possible will cause the fire to burn through the night. This is a safe, constant, moderate heat fire with low light and a long burning time. When combined with a heat reflector, it is capable of a much higher amount of heat radiation.

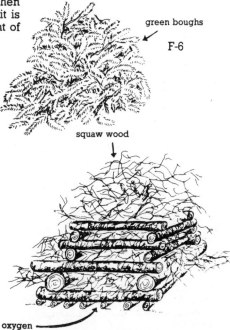

green boughs

F-6

squaw wood

oxygen

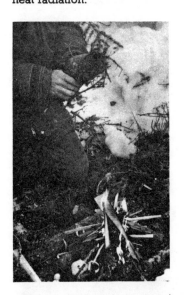

Figure # F-6 is your signal fire. It is always built pyramid style because you want a fast, large, hot fire. For night-time use you want the light and for day time use you will want smoke. Your smoke will be achieved by a well established pyramid fire made from very dry squaw wood (small dead spruce or pine branches). After your signal fire has been lit and is really burning well, pile enough green boughs on it so as to suffocate the fire (stop its oxygen flow). This will result in a heavy column of smoke that can be seen for miles. This will be covered in depth in the chapter on signaling.

21

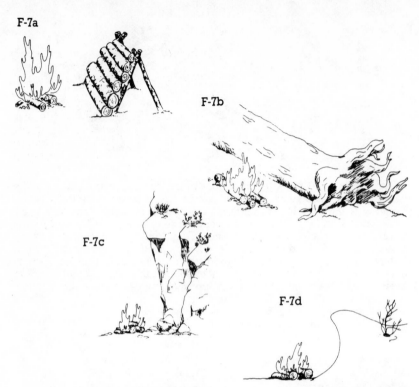

F-7a

F-7b

F-7c

F-7d

Figure # F-7 covers some different forms of fire reflectors. Their purpose is to re-radiate heat normally lost, back in your direction. They are effective and if stone is used, you have created a heat sink which will store and re-radiate heat to you even after the fire has gone out. If logs are used, they should be large and of green wood. The use of a reflector will without a doubt, increase the amount of heat radiated in your direction with less fuel. More on this will be covered in the sheltering chapter. The reflector can also serve as a fine clothes drying rack, etc.

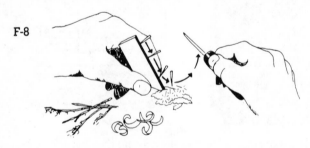

F-8

Figure # F-8 shows the proper way of using your flint and what is very important here is that your have all your fire building materials already gathered and close at hand. As you know, once you have ignited your primary fire starter you must have tinder and very small kindling ready to add to the small fire. As the fire grows so will the size of your kindling and final fuel.

F-9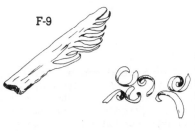

Figure # F-9 illustrates feather sticks, and curly cues. They make excellent fuel after the first small flame is created from your fire starter and/or fine tinder. Once the feather sticks and tinder has started to burn you can carefully add slightly larger, dry kindling. Be careful not to smother (cut off oxygen supply) the fire. At this point more dry, larger fuel can be added. You now have a fire and larger wood should be placed carefully on it. If you are in a situation where most of the wood you have gathered is wet, place it near the fire to dry out. At this time dry some tinder and kindling for tomorrow's fire.

F-10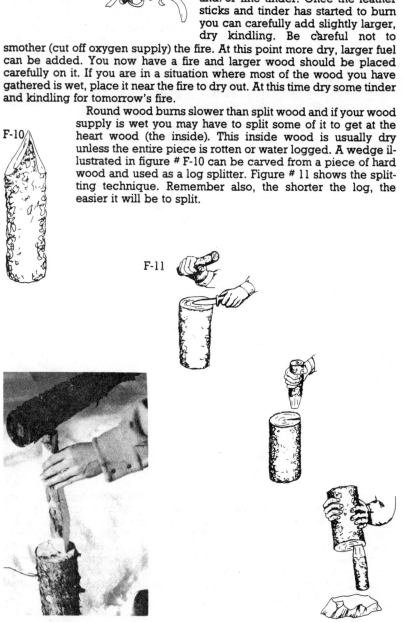

Round wood burns slower than split wood and if your wood supply is wet you may have to split some of it to get at the heart wood (the inside). This inside wood is usually dry unless the entire piece is rotten or water logged. A wedge illustrated in figure # F-10 can be carved from a piece of hard wood and used as a log splitter. Figure # 11 shows the splitting technique. Remember also, the shorter the log, the easier it will be to split.

F-11

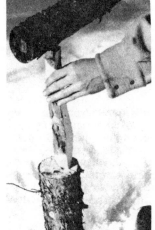

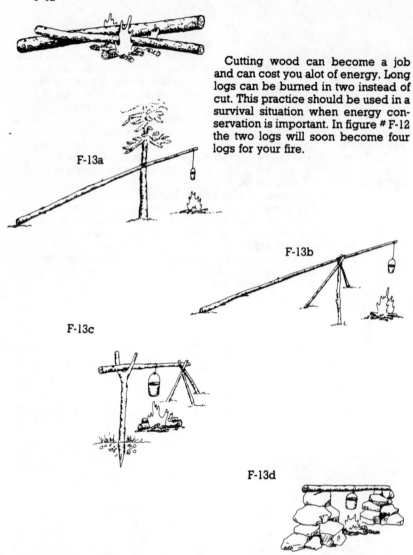

Cutting wood can become a job and can cost you alot of energy. Long logs can be burned in two instead of cut. This practice should be used in a survival situation when energy conservation is important. In figure # F-12 the two logs will soon become four logs for your fire.

F-13a

F-13b

F-13c

F-13d

Now that you have a good fire and it's already working for you, a few things should be added to make life easier and more comfortable for you. In figure # F-13 you will find various types of cooking poles and apparatus. I find the swing pole my favorite and the most versatile. It can be rotated horizontally and vertically with very littel effort to accomodate many different duties and fires. When I am deciding exactly where I intend to build my shelter and fire, I try to choose a suitable location that has a small standing tree to attach the pole to. If this in not possible, I use one of the alternative variations.

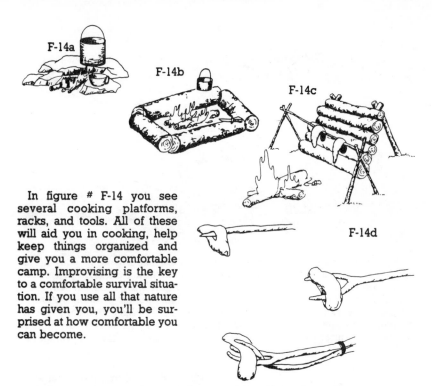

F-14a

F-14b

F-14c

F-14d

In figure # F-14 you see several cooking platforms, racks, and tools. All of these will aid you in cooking, help keep things organized and give you a more comfortable camp. Improvising is the key to a comfortable survival situation. If you use all that nature has given you, you'll be surprised at how comfortable you can become.

In figure # F-15 you see two types of improvised stoves. The first one, # F-15a is using a discarded can to burn any kind of oil, whether it be from the crankcase of an engine or animal fat. Make your wick from cloth, rope, string, etc. Fasten it to a holder made from wire, a green stick, or anything that will support it and not burn too readily. Give the wick a few minutes to soak up some of the oil in the container and then light it. This type of stove will burn similarly to a kerosene lamp and will give heat and light in a small shelter.

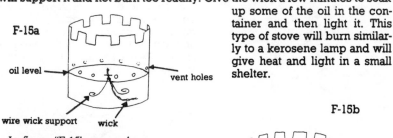

F-15a

oil level

vent holes

wire wick support   wick

F-15b

In figure #F-15b we are burning fuel oil or gasoline. There is no wick here and the sand acts as a catalyst. With this stove as well as the one in figure # F-15a, small oxygen holes must be punched in the area of the base of the flame. Flow-through ventilation must be allowed at the top especially if it is to be covered with a cooking pan, can, or pot.

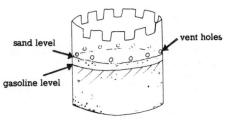

sand level

vent holes

gasoline level

25

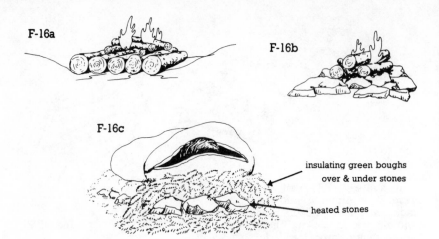

F-16a

F-16b

F-16c

insulating green boughs
over & under stones

heated stones

Fire platforms as shown in figure # F-16a are used to keep your fire off very wet ground, deep snow, or ice. By using such a platform you will be able to build a fire with an extremely unfavorable base location. If wood is used, it must be green and as large in diameter as possible. Stone, if available, works very well. Stones can be heated in this fashion and also by placing them near and around the fire. These heated stones can then be moved to your shelter sleeping area to act as a radiant heater (See figure # F-16c).

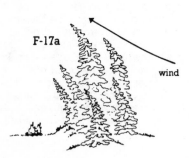

F-17a

wind

Figure # F-17 shows the importance of properly controlled draft, that is, the amount of oxygen getting to the fire. We discussed earlier how important this oxygen flow is to keep your fire burning but now you can see that too much forced oxygen will cause your fire to burn too rapidly, use too much fuel, cast sparks everywhere, and can smoke you out. Your fire should always be built out of the wind so you have control over it.

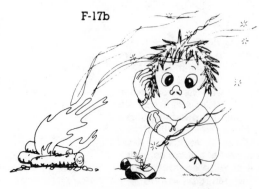

F-17b

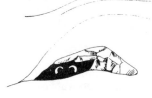

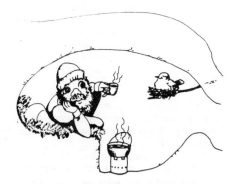

CHAPTER #5
Sheltering

As Webster states, a shelter is something that covers, protects, or someplace affording protection, as from the elements, danger, etc. Shelter implies the protection of something that covers, as a roof or other structure that shields one from the elements, danger, etc.

In wilderness survival, your shelter will serve one or several of the following purposes:

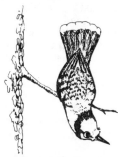

* Protection from the cold
* Protection from the rain
* Protection from the wind
* Protection from insects
* Protection from snow
* Protection from too much sun

Shelters can be built in their entirety from mother nature's warehouse if necessary. But shelter building becomes much easier if you have a few items in a well planned survival kit. We will discuss both approaches in this chapter.

My first three choices of the most important materials and tools to have with me for sheltering would be:

* A knife
* Nylon cord
* A good survival saw

With these three items you can be very comfortable in a survival situation as far as shelter building. A very important fact to remember here is no matter how many or how few tools you have to work with, keep track of them; never just lay them around, and don't abuse them. They are all you have to work with, and they may mean your life or death.

If you have decided to stay in one spot and wait for rescue, which in most cases I strongly advise, you should build a shelter. In the survival kits we give our students, shelters and shelter-making materials are included to build a shelter under any geological or climactic condition.

This makes shelter-building easy, which again conserves precious energy. In the kit is a special one-man tent (but which can sleep two) with floor and bug screen. This is ideal for the summer, and only takes minutes to set up. There is also a piece of rip-stop nylon that measures 8' X 8' with sewn-in reinforcements and nylon tie downs. This piece of cloth is extremely useful if you know how and when to use it.

Also in the kit is nylon parachute cord. I like to have 150' but only 85' is required. This nylon cord is one of the most useful survival tools you can have. If you are making up your own kit don't cheat on the nylon cord, and don't take more than 150'. That's all you will need, and any more will just take up valuable room and add needless weight to your kit.

The next item you should have is a saw of some kind. Be careful if you are buying a survival saw. There are a lot of saws on the market that look nice but are inefficient when it comes to cutting wood. The best by far for its size, is the Air Force Survival saw/machete/snow shovel combination tool which is part of my larger kit.

A small folding saw that will cut meat and bone, as well as wood, is the Sierra Saw. I feel these two saws compliment each other and should both be in your large kit. Bear in mind, my kit and the kits I make for students measure approximately 16" X 12" X 16". Half of that is a break-away medical kit. With the proper planning and knowledge, you can and will have a kit with every item you need. You can do with less but your knowledge must be much greater and more energy will be used in your survival tasks.

The first question is what kind of shelter shall you build? The determining factors that will answer this question are: terrain, natural resources available, weather, and snow conditions. These factors will tell you exactly what kind of shelter to build. What you are about to do now is the area where most people fail. Instead of trying to fight nature (a losing battle) you are going to become in harmony with it and even take it one step further and let nature work for you.

In the following examples pretend you were in an airplane which has just crashed and you have some minor injuries. Your first move is to attend to these minor injuries so you can keep them minor. This is no problem because your first aid kit has everything you need in it. Now that has been accomplished, you are going to set up camp for the first night. In order of priority, you must have water, shelter & fire.

Example # 1 - You are down in an area with few trees, mostly brush, three feet of snow, no visable rivers or lakes, and it's 40° below zero. Things look grim; or do they? You already know what is going against you, so let's look at what's in your favor and what kind of shelter you are going to build. Let's run down what's around you again. #1 - we have an inoperable aircraft that has a wealth of survival materials in it. It has a storage of gasoline which you already know can be a fuel source. It has a crankcase full of oil, again a heat source. But remember the temperature—it's 40° below and that oil should be drained into a container now, before it gets too thick. The foam rubber in the seats makes excellent fuel, especially if soaked in oil.

Fabric in the seats may make fine wicks for a home-made lamp or small oil stove. Things don't look quite so grim; you've got a hardware store right in front of you and, your survival kit at your side. Next you look around and are certain that there are few but enough trees to build an A-Frame. There is a lot of snow which means an endless supply of pure water and the main material to build your shelter out of. Remember the aircraft will not be your shelter. It will soon become an ice box.

Let's see what we have at this point. We have fire-making materials, shelter-making materials, water, and a huge signal already made for us—the aircraft. In this case you are in good shape with everything but food. So this will be your next move after proper signaling has been set-up. Things now look good for you and the A-Frame snow shelter is your choice.

Example # 2—You are down in a spruce forest, it's winter, one foot of snow, it's 60° below zero. As you look around you already know parts of the aircraft are useable, there are trees everywhere and they are fuel for you and a frame for your shelter. There is enough snow for your water supply. It's deadly cold, but with these temperatures comes dryness, so with a little care you won't be getting wet. A spruce forest means food, both plant and animal. Again, you are going to be O.K. and your shelter will be snow covered lean-to or A-Frame.

Examples # 3—You are down in the arctic above the tree line with no trees or shrubs available, it's 30° below with winds of 35 mph, several feet of snow cover on the ground. The wind that has given you a chill factor of −100° (flesh can freeze in 30 seconds) has also made your shelter for you. As the wind shifts and moves the snow, it becomes very hard. Your choice of shelters will be a snow cave or snow trench and once inside this type of shelter, regardless of the outside wind or temperature, you will be in a safe, wind-free environment of between 22 degrees and 28 degrees above zero, or even higher depending on your skills, and needs at the time.

Example # 4—You've just gone down in a spruce forest, it's 65° degrees above zero, the mosquitoes and no-see-ums are intolerable. Your shelter at this time can be the aircraft or the small screened survival tent in your kit.

In these four examples, I have covered a wide range of terrain and temperature conditions that could be encountered in the north. I will be referring back to these examples in this and following chapters. As you can see at this point, nature will almost always give you a shelter or a means of making one. You should always take full advantage of this to help you on your way to staying safe and being rescued.

I remember one time when Gretchen, my wife and co-director of our survival institute, and I were doing research on an island on the southern Alaska coast. Everything went as planned until weather made pick-up impossible for almost two weeks after it was scheduled. When pick-up finally came we were so well established on the island that we hated to leave.

So, a survival experience doesn't have to be a horror show. It can often be even pleasant if you make it so.

You can improvise a shelter from the natural materials in your vicinity, use parts from your aircraft, ATV, or car, and if you choose to travel with one of my survival kits or a kit you have made personally, sheltering is no problem. The kind of shelter you choose will depend on the ambient temperature, the terrain, material resources, and insects. Your campsite should be selected carefully and you should always try to be close to your fuel and water supply. Both are very important and dehydration is every bit as much of a killer as hypothermia.

Your shelter will have to guard you from insects and rain. You'll want to pick a site that affords a breeze, in dry ground, and out of the deep woods that is infested with insects, if possible. Insects can't fly in a good breeze, so nature is working for you if you take advantage of it. Don't sleep on bare ground; nature provides a tremendous amount of ground insulating materials like spruce or pine boughs, dry grass, leaves or thoroughly dried moss. For summer use I prefer a lean-to because of its room. In the kit that I carry is enough mosquito netting to seal it off. If I'm on the move I use the small special tent also in the kit or build a simple A-Frame and use the nylon cloth and bug screen.

When assembling the frame work for your shelter you should always cut the smallest possible wood that will still do the job adequately. If you use oversized wood you will use more energy than necessary, your lashings will require more cord, and you will find yourself soon running out of energy and materials. I find that working with wood two inches in diameter and smaller works well, but that depends on the materials and tools available. Frame work should be kept simple but strong, and built in a dry location.

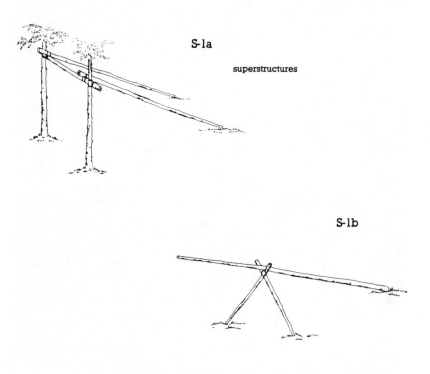

S-1a

superstructures

S-1b

As you can see from the figures S-2a and S-2b, your shelter can be erected with vertical or horizontal frame work. In all cases I have found that horizontal frame work is superior because the covering layer of spruce boughs attaches much easier. The only disadvantage is it takes more lashing and longer pieces of wood. If the materials are available, this is the way to go. If not, the vertical framework is a good alternative. Again, let mother nature tell you what to do; listen and survive.

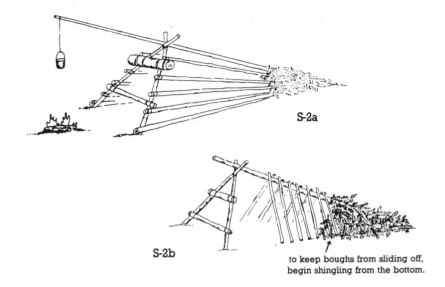

S-2a

S-2b

to keep boughs from sliding off,
begin shingling from the bottom.

In all shelters of this kind the superstructure (your first poles) must be the largest and strongest. All the rest of your shelter materials will rest on these. I also recommend that on any lean-to, a sitting pole be built (see figure # S-4a). It is a comfortable way to sit off the ground and puts you right in front of the fire. It's only one more piece of wood and in my estimation, it's worth it. It also doubles as an equipment hanging rack and a clothes drying rack. A good point can be brought up here about your equipment; it is limited, so do not scatter it. Consolidate it in one spot or you will lose it. When I'm building a shelter I always build an equipment rack even if it's temporary so I don't lose my tools. **NEVER** lay anything on the ground away from your shelter or you will lose it.

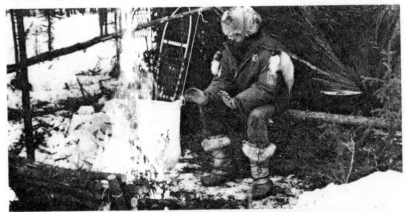

After you have decided what kind of shelter you will build and have picked your location you should build a fire where it's going to be permanent. Have your fire going while you are building the shelter. This is important because as you build you are using a great amount of water in your body that must be replenished during the building process. Whether it be summer or winter, you need water replacement right away. So get your fire go-

31

ing and start either generating water, or purifyng it. Either way you must drink as much as you can. We will cover water procurement in depth in a following chapter, but for now remember, start your shelter building after you have started a fire and have some sort of water process going.

As you start your shelter, the way you lash is important. Three wraps and three fraps give you the maximum strength of the nylon cord, any more is a waste of materials you can't afford. The following illustration shows, in detail, the method you should use. Remember, less than three wraps makes your shelter weaker and more is a waste. The superstructure should be done this way along with the sitting pole. The rest you can cheat on with no adverse affects (See figure # S-3a-c).

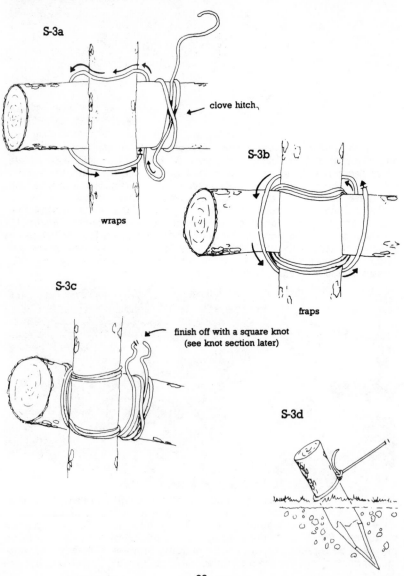

S-3a

clove hitch

S-3b

wraps

S-3c

fraps

finish off with a square knot
(see knot section later)

S-3d

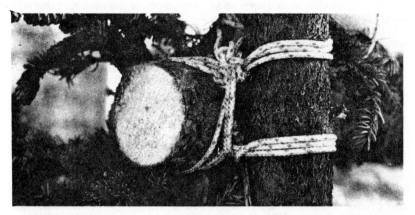

I always use spruce boughs, if available, in a crisscrossed, almost woven manner, as a floor of my lean-to or A-Frame. They insulate me from the ground, and are extremely comfortable. As you are building your shelter always drag the whole tree to the shelter before knocking off the boughs. This way, when your frame work is complete, you will be surrounded with boughs to use for the shelter top and floor without having to hunt for them, again saving valuable energy. Whenever possible, fashion a club to knock the boughs off. It is by far the easiest way to clean the boughs from a spruce tree. And if by chance you hit yourself with the club, the injury won't be nearly as severe as if you were using a machete or axe.

Once you have your superstructure erected, it's time to put your spruce boughs in place. If you have chosen horizontal framework, this will be an easy task. Completely cover the shelter with the boughs, both top and sides. From your kit take out the nylon cloth and cover this framework and your wind, and rain resistant shelter is almost finished. Without the survival kit's cloth, the more boughs the better.

I have come up with a fine compliment to the lean-to out of our kits. On the underside of the lean-to roof or A-Frame, lash your survival blankets. They make the shelter water proof, and reflect a tremendous amount of heat. Also, one blanket goes under you when you sleep to insure moisture protection. If insects are a problem, your mosquito net is put across the front next. You now have a fine shelter, a warm fire, and water. Tomorrow your first job is to set up your signals and then start on food procurement.

Your winter shelter will have to protect you from the cold and that will definitely be your first consideration.

If little or no snow is available you are going to need a good fuel source, and if there is no snow you will want to be camping near a water supply. I would suggest under these conditions either a lean-to or a double lean-to. A double lean-to can be kept warmer with less fuel because the fire is inside. You'll have to make the choice at the time. Both shelters work very well and afford plenty of room for both you and your equipment.

You can also build an A-Frame which will take fewer materials and work, but your room inside will be much less. If you are going to be on the move, the A-Frame will be your choice.

If snow is available make use of it. It is a fine insulator. Snow will be your source of water but never eat snow. You must melt it first.

A single lean-to is easy to build and can be a summer or winter shelter. When built properly this shelter will shed rain, keep out flying insects, help keep you warm, and keep snow off of you and your equipment. The summer shelter is shown in this figure. If you have no tools or nylon cord, the single lean-to can still be built.

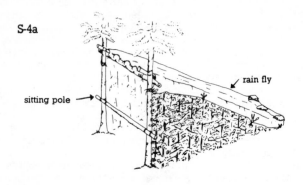

S-4a

rain fly

sitting pole →

When building this type of lean-to your fire should be directly in front of it and a reflector on the far side of the fire. This will reflect an ample amount of heat back to the lean-to, and trap more inside. Heat retention will be better if the inside of the shelter is lined with foil survival blankets. Your floor should be covered with spruce or pine boughs to give you a comfortable, dry sleeping area. If stones are available they can be heated by the fire and placed inside your shelter for even more heat and flat heated stones can be placed directly under your sleeping area and covered with more spruce boughs to protect you from being burned.

After the superstructure and secondary structure have been completed, the framework can be covered with a piece of plastic, or nylon material if available. The nylon works well but the plastic will keep the shelter completely water proof even in a pouring rain.

If you decide to build a front-canopy-extension type lean-to, it will help you keep away flying insects and will keep your fire from the rain. This addition will make your quarters a little smokey but that is what you are trying to achieve, because the smoke will drive away the flying insects.

All in all, the single lean-to is a good choice of shelters and should always be considered. It's roomy, comfortable, and moderately warm.

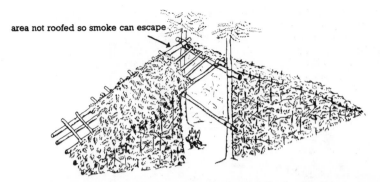

area not roofed so smoke can escape

The double lean-to is illustrated in figure # 2-4b. It affords a tremendous amount of room and it becomes a warmer and more permanent shelter. It has the fire inside so there is less heat loss to the outside. This is not just an overnight shelter because of the length of time it takes to build. If you plan to spend a long time in one location, serious consideration should be given to this type of shelter.

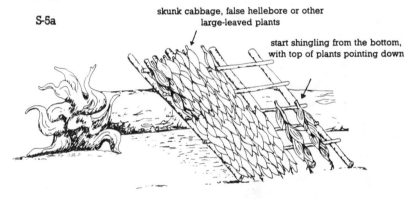

S-5a

skunk cabbage, false hellebore or other large-leaved plants

start shingling from the bottom, with top of plants pointing down

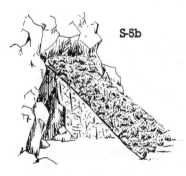

S-5b

Figures # S-5a & b show different modifications and variations of the standard lean-to. Whenever nature has done half your work for you, you should take advantage of it. I have spent more nights in the modified lean-to than in the conventional style just because they are easier to build and this saves time and energy.

A-Frames are illustrated in figures # S-2a and S-2b. This is a good shelter but has limited inside space. It can be erected quickly with fewer materials than a lean-to. This is a good overnight choice and can be used in summer or winter.

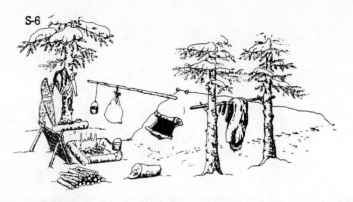

Figure # S-6 shows how a well organized camp can and should be built. Everything has its place, and the wilderness has become a comfortable place to live. This type of camp gives you a good psychological foundation, keeps your tools and materials from being lost or broken and is efficient, which means you will burn fewer calories.

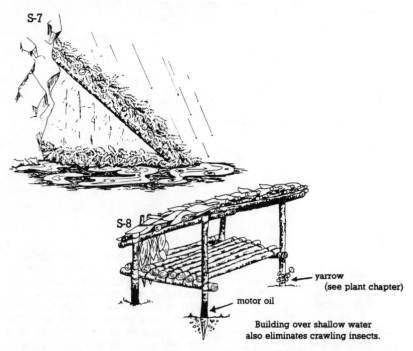

yarrow
(see plant chapter)

motor oil

Building over shallow water
also eliminates crawling insects.

Figures # S-7 and S-8 both show raised shelters. Their purpose is to get you off the gound level, either because of a water problem, or because of crawling insects such as ants. In most cases, the water problem can be solved by more spruce boughs on the floor of the shelter. A good example of this is one time when Gretchen and I were camping in the winter in a very remote area and, because of the snow conditions, decided to dig in. To get to the ground we had to go about five feet down. We covered this shelter with a roof and chose to use a fire inside, using the snow wall as a reflector. This worked very well but as could be expected, the snow wall did some melting. Our sleeping quarters stayed dry because of the deep bed of spruce boughs we used on the floor. Any water ran underneath and we stayed dry and warm.

When using these types of raised shelters for crawling insect control, the effectiveness can be increased by wiping the leg sections with oil if available, as from the crankcase of a disabled vehecle or by wiping them with yarrow, one of many plants that is a natural insect repellent. After I wipe the legs, I tie some of the whole plant on each leg. Again nature has given us what we need, all we have to do is use it. The yarrow can be rubbed directly on the skin for one of nature's natural insect repellants.

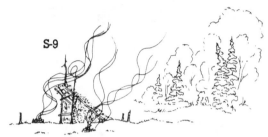

S-9

When sheltering-in and flying insects are a problem you should, as I have already mentioned, stay out of the deep woods if possible. This is where the insects thrive and will be in their greatest numbers. If you can, build your shelter where there is plenty of sunlight and a breeze and the flying insects will not be as concentrated. If necessary, build your fire (or in extreme cases, fires) so as to be almost always getting some smoke around you. Use small fires with green or rotten, damp wood and you will have plenty of smoke.

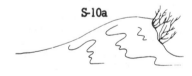

S-10a

Your choice of snow shelter location will dictate the type of shelter and how much energy you will have to expend building it. The amount and type of snow is very important. Take a few minutes to survey the area and nature again will tell you what to do. For instance, if there is an area that is subject to windy conditions the snow will be constantly drifting and building up in depth and firmness. In an area like this you can simply tunnel in because nature has already made the snow deep and hard. Whenever snow is moved or worked, either by wind or by you, it will set up and harden similar to mortar. So if the wind has already done the job for you, take advantage of it.

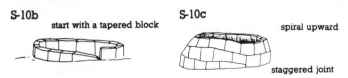

S-10b
start with a tapered block

S-10c
spiral upward

staggered joint

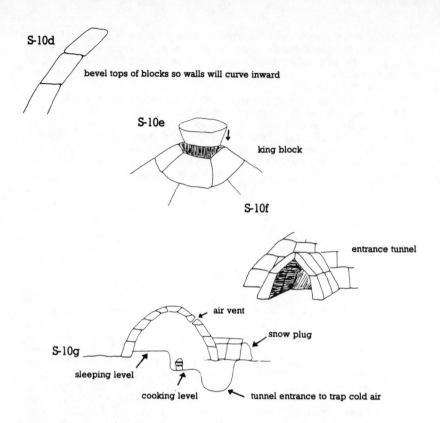

S-10d

bevel tops of blocks so walls will curve inward

S-10e

king block

S-10f

entrance tunnel

air vent

snow plug

S-10g

sleeping level

cooking level

tunnel entrance to trap cold air

Knowing that this area has hard snow, it is a choice place to cut snow blocks if you choose to build a shelter similar to an igloo. Snow block shelters work extremely well and can be constructed fairly quickly. They can also afford you alot of room. If nature provides you with the hard snow and you plan to stay in this location for some time, this is probably the way to go. Building the igloo is not hard but requires practice. Make a winter game out of it with your family. It will make a fine play house for the children when you are done.

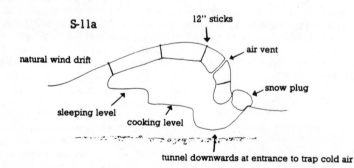

S-11a

12" sticks

air vent

natural wind drift

snow plug

sleeping level

cooking level

tunnel downwards at entrance to trap cold air

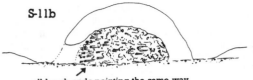

S-11b

all brush ends pointing the same way
so they can be removed through a small doorway

S-11c

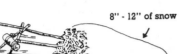

8" - 12" of snow

green boughs over framework

In figure # S-11 you will see the construction of the three major snow caves that are commonly used. All three work well. In a shelter such as figure # S-11a, you tunnel into a snow bank that the wind has made for you. Remember when building with snow always try to end up with at least 10" to 12" of snow for insulation and strength. This can be gauged very easily by inserting small sticks 12" long from the outside at random points in the area where you plan to tunnel. As you start hollowing your cave ceiling out and you come to a stick end, you know you still have 12" of cover at that point and you will stop digging there. Soon all the stick points will appear and you can be assured of nice thick 12" walls. Wherever possible try to build a sleeping shelf. Cold air settles to the floor and you will be warmer, at this higher level.

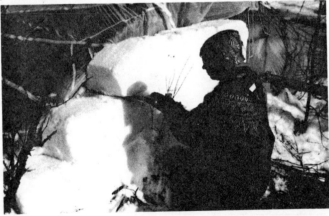

In figure # S-11b, you are working with a limited amount of snow on the ground so you must scrape the snow from under the cave location and from around it. In this type of construction you will first clear the area where the cave is to be built and fill this area with a pile of small spruce trees and brush the size you want the inside of your shelter to be. If possible cover this brush with a tarp or cloth of some kind. Next start working the snow, constantly rolling it toward the cave and start piling it on the brush heap. Also make sure all the brush is lying in the same direction. Once you have covered the entire pile of brush with about 12" of worked and rolled snow you must leave it alone for a few hours. Test it by touch every once in a while, until it has set up like concrete. Once this happens, make as small an entrance as possible at the end nearest the bases of the pieces of brush and start gently pulling out pieces of brush one at a time. Soon all of the brush will be removed and your cave will be finished except for laying spruce boughs on the floor and making a snow plug for the door entrance.

No matter what kind of snow cave you are building the entrance should be fitted well with a snow plug. A snow plug is either a block of snow cut to size or even better, a piece of cloth filled with snow. This second type of plug is easier to use and easier to handle. Take your cloth, lay it on the ground and put a pile of snow in the center. Then fold up all the corners and tie them together. Bounce this bag of snow on the ground several times to work it so it will set up. You will next fit it into your snow cave entrance opening, and leave it there to harden. Once it has hardened into shape it can be removed and stored for when you will need it. When you enter the cave all you need do is pull the plug, "bag of snow", part way in behind you.

Illustration S-11c shows an A-Frame snow cave. This cave is built similarly to the one in figure # S-11b, except it has a permanent, standing superstructure (inside framework). The A-Frame is built as shown after the snow has been cleaned from the ground area. One very important thing to remember when constructing this type of snow shelter is that a relatively large log must be placed over the entrance to support the snow over it. This is shown in the illustration.

S-12a

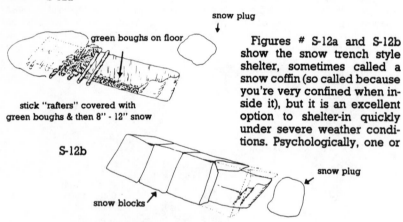

snow plug

green boughs on floor

stick "rafters" covered with green boughs & then 8" - 12" snow

S-12b

snow blocks

snow plug

Figures # S-12a and S-12b show the snow trench style shelter, sometimes called a snow coffin (so called because you're very confined when inside it), but it is an excellent option to shelter-in quickly under severe weather conditions. Psychologically, one or

two nights will be as much as you probably will want to spend in this shelter. This is a temporary shelter but very effective for keeping you alive when it's deadly cold. It is usually my choice when I'm on the move in extremely cold weather conditions.

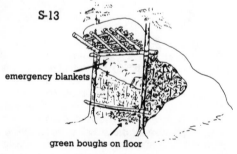

S-13

emergency blankets

green boughs on floor

40

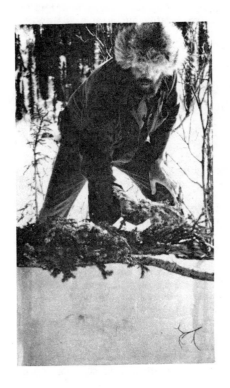

In figure # S-13, you see the lean-to again but this time it is insulated with snow. It's a very roomy and comfortable type of shelter but you will need plenty of fuel for your fire to keep it warm. Under severe cold weather conditions the single lean-to will not be warm enough but a double lean-to will work well.

Important Things to Remember

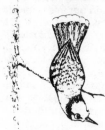

* When building a snow cave, the more you work the snow (move it around) the faster and harder it will set up.
* All snow caves and igloos must have a vent or air hole (preferably cut in at a 45° angle) especially if you use any kind of internal heat source such as a candle or improvised stove.
* Pick a snow cave location close to a good supply of snow. Moving snow is hard work and a drain on precious energy reserves.

* When using wood framework for your shelter use smaller diameter poles to make less work.
* Always take the time to survey the area you plan to shelter in and think what is best for that particular situation.
* Try to keep 10" to 12" of snow cover on any snow shelter or cave.
* When summer sheltering, insects can be a very real problem. Remember flying insects do not like wind, smoke, and certain natural plants like yarrow.
* Always protect yourself from underneath with spruce boughs or some other insulation from cold and dampness.
* Never build a shelter under anything that may fall on it and injure you.
* When building near water make sure you are always above high water mark or high tide mark.
* When building your shelter, especially in cold weather, you must take off enough clothes to compensate for the warming caused by physical activity. If you don't, your clothing will become wet with perspiration and you will be a candidate for hypothermia.
* Always try to expend as little energy as possible while setting up camp. Try to be close to the source of fuel for your fire.
* Start generating and drinking water right away and consume as much as you can. Dehydration is a killer.
* Build an organizing area or shelf to keep track of your survival equipment and tools.
* Never lay a tool down anywhere it might get covered with snow, etc. and be lost.
* Never be in a rush. When you hurry, accidents and mistakes happen.
* Always let nature work for you; don't try to fight it. Become in harmony with your surroundings.

CHAPTER # 6
Food Procurment - Fishing

Food procurement will fall under 4 major categories: fish, plants, mammals, and birds. From these you will get all your nourishment to sustain life and maintain good health. This can be a fulfulling experience and almost all of these food sources not only contain what you need but can be delicious. Each year I harvest food from all four categories to make up the major part of my diet. The price is right, it's enjoyable, it's good for me, and good-tasting.

When in an extended wilderness survival situation you will have some or all of these food sources to choose from. Nature has given you a store house of food and it is up to you to recognize and harvest it. This should be done with as little effort as possible. You never want to expend more energy procuring food than you will receive from it. A good example are any bears that for one reason or another come out of their dens too early in the spring and are confronted with cold temperatures and deep snow. They attempt to find food but being poorly adapted to travel in deep snow, expend many calories without finding enough food to replace them. So they return to their dens and almost all inevitably die of starvation while they sleep. The bears that come out from their dens at the appropriate time of the year have little trouble moving under the conditions that they are adapted to (little or no snow) and easily find sufficient food to maintain their calorie reserve. Here again we can learn an important lesson from nature, the master instructor.

This simple mathematical balance is: outgo of calories of energy can not exceed the intake. As soon as fat and energy reserves are depleted, death results-always, just like when your car runs out of fuel. It stops no matter what, because its energy source has been completely exhausted. During severe weather conditions, birds & mammals are not out expending energy, they know to live with nature and not fight it, so they wait the storms out and conserve the priceless energy they have until food procurement becomes easy for them. The animals are the teachers, we are the students. When food is abundant, gather it, enjoy it, and store as much as you can because tomorrow nature may change things.

First let us talk about fish. They live in one form or another almost everywhere in the world where there is water. If your situation leaves you in an area where there is water containing fish, you have an excellent source of food. You'll be getting protein, minerals & vitamins, but remember anything you cook will lose most of its vitamin C and certain B vitamins after exposure to heat. These you must get from other sources. If you've found a good area to fish, your only other problem is how to get them out of the water and into the pan. Running up and down a stream and thrashing about is surely not the answer. Besides being unproductive, you are bound to get wet, tired, and you certainly will burn up calories at a rapid rate.

Don't laugh, sometimes when people are lost and hungry they may do crazy things. My advice is to sit down for a while, rest, look at the water, watch the animals and birds around and in it, and learn from what you see.

After sitting awhile and watching that lake or river, what might you see? Remember what I teach at the institute is not a hit or miss chance of survival but a proven system that will work every time if you let it. First of all, if you see no plant life in a lake, you are watching the wrong lake. If no plants are present, there will be limited or no oxygen present in the water. Without oxygen there will be no fish, and if there are no fish you would be wasting your time and energy to fish it.

Next, I would look closely to see if there were any small invertebrates of any kind, including aquatic insects. If this search proved again negative I would not only depart from the lake but under no circumstances, drink any of the water. As you can see the water itself can show you many secrets, but you must look and see them.

Now lets look at a similar lake. While you sit there relaxed and very still, you see alot of aquatic plant life. Wait a minute, you see one reed move, then another and another, in a straight line in rapid succession out to the deep water. What you probably just witnessed was a member of the pike family getting his dinner. Pike, being a predator fish, like to lie near the edge of weeded areas, the weeds offering them camouflage as they wait for a smaller fish to swim by in the open.

Before we go any further on how to read the lake, we should note that since there is a good chance what you saw was a pike of some sort, and if so, your food source is close. What's really important at this time is that you remember that a pike, especially the northern pike, can attain considerable size and has a mouth full of teeth that will cut your line. In this case you will want to use a wire leader between the bait and line. It only has to be 6" to 8" long but it will save you losing your lure. In my kits I furnish a wire leader and a red and white daredevil spoon. This is the combination you should use. Cast the lure out into deep water, try to keep it off the bottom and retrieve it through large openings in the weeds if possible. If pike are present, get ready for a very fast and forceful strike, a good fight, and a fine dinner (see figures # P-1 and P-2).

P-1

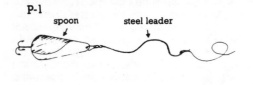

spoon   steel leader

P-2   cast to here

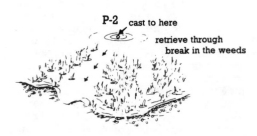

retrieve through
break in the weeds

As you sit and watch the lake, take notice of any animal activity, a muskrat for instance. Besides being a delicious taste treat himself, he spends all his life gathering food and storing it in feeding stations (mounds of cut plant life shaped like little domes) here and there on the lake in fairly shallow water. The contents of these mounds is a very good food source to consider because a muskrat is very selective in what he harvests and anything he eats is edible for you. And he has it stored right in front of you by the ton (see figure # P-3).

P-3

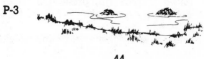

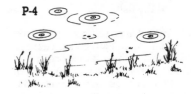

P-4

Take note of the types of food the muskrat is storing so you can recognize them growing in their natural state. Then you already know at least one edible wild plant in your area. In the winter of course, you will have to rely on the food the muskrat has already stored for you.

As you continue to watch the lake, you may see beaver, with habits similar to the muskrat, or a certain kind of shore bird, or maybe ducks and geese. A close investigation of the shallow water may reveal freshwater mussels and edible aquatic plants. Now that you are reading and understanding the lake, you might as well catch that pike; he's waiting for the lure.

While you are preparing dinner and relaxing afterwards, keep your eyes on that lake and it wouldn't hurt to take a short walk along it. Watch the surface and if there are several water rings in it from fish coming to the surface feeding on insects, especially in early evening, you are probably watching trout or grayling feeding (see figure # P-4). So tomorrow night you might try some dry flies in that area when they are feeding and have a change of diet to trout or grayling. Remember if you see them feeding on the surface, fish the surface. If possible get a good look at the insects that will be all over the water and try to match your fly as closely as possible to those insects. All the answers are there; all you have to do is look.

During your evening walk, constantly be checking the shore for tracks of the small and larger mammals that are frequenting your lake. Do not make your evening camp anywhere near an area where there are several sets of bear tracks. You're full now, you've had some exercise and it's time for a good night's sleep. Tomorrow you will be busy collecting edible plants, setting out your snares, and fishing. If there are fish in the lake you'll want to start catching every one you can and smoking and drying them for later use. Almost all animals store food and it should be a lesson for you.

P-5

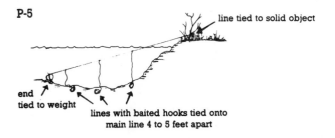

line tied to solid object

end tied to weight

lines with baited hooks tied onto main line 4 to 5 feet apart

P-6

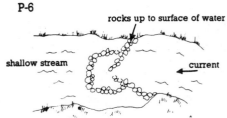

rocks up to surface of water

shallow stream

current

Most lakes have some form of bottom feeding fish in them. For these you can put out set-lines and using the entrails of fish you caught during the day for bait, let the bottom fish catch themselves for you while you sleep (see figure # P-5). If you find sizable fish in fairly shallow water you can spear

45

them. You can build a trap in streams and herd the fish into it like cattle (see figure # P-6).

If you have a gill net or the means to make one, it is an extremely effective method of taking fish. And last but not least, you can poison them. There are a number of plants that when crushed and mixed with water to form a thick liquid and added to a stream or lake, will kill every fish that comes in contact with it. In my kits I carry one of these, taken from the derris plant. When premixed with a little water and then distributed in a stream, (only one ounce and a 12% solution) will kill all the fish for at least ½ a mile down stream in a creek that is betwwen 20 and 30 feet wide. It's quite impressive, I would advise assembling a trap down stream to save you work and fish. The warmer the water the faster it acts, but even in cooler water it is effective. In water below 50 degrees it starts to become ineffective. Lime put in small ponds or tidal pools will kill with equal effectiveness. Lime will be the end product of burned sea shells, coral, limestone, etc.

Remember that almost any method of taking sport fish other than rod and reel, is considered illegal in most places, so it shouldn't be done for fun. But in a true survival situation, staying alive is your primary concern. When its your life at stake you make the rules and regulations. As a friend of mine once said jokingly, if you're ever lost and need help, commit a fish or game violation and surely a fish or game warden will appear.

Fishing Tips

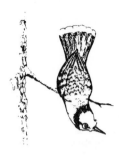

* When fishing in weedy areas always test for pike first with a spoon and wire leader. They have sharp teeth and can cut a normal fishing line.
* If you've caught a pike, be careful on removing the hook. Do not put your fingers in his mouth.
* To remove the hook and control the pike, hold him with your thumb in one eye and a finger in the other (this will paralize the fish).
* If fish are feeding on the surface of a lake or stream you also should fish the surface with dry flies.

* If fish are present but not biting on your lure, change styles and/or color of lure. Fish strike for one of three reasons: because of hunger, fear, or protectiveness. By choosing the right type and color lure you can make them strike.
* An eye from a previously caught fish will make excellent bait on a hook, especially when fishing through the ice.
* The more erratic the action of your lure, the more likely a strike.
* Whenever you can use natural bait, do so.
* Do not use too big of a hook for the type of fish you are trying to catch. It is better to have too small of a hook than too large.
* All knots tied in your line should be carefully done. They will be the weakest part of your line.
* When fishing with a jig constantly bounce it off the bottom.
* When you get a strike, set the hook with a firm tug.
* When bringing in the fish, keep tension on the line at all times and keep the rod tip high.
* Improvise a gaff hook (one is included in my kit) and use it to remove the fish from the water (see figure # P-7).

P-8

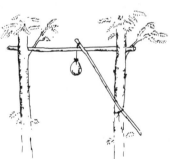

P-7

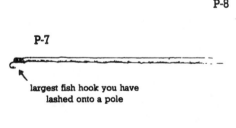

largest fish hook you have
lashed onto a pole

pick a spot not close to your camp

* Always remember how you were fishing when you get a strike, and continue with that method. It worked once and probably will again.
* If you are not catching fish change your methods or lures (some fish like a fast retrieve and some like it very slow).
* Always save eyes and entrails for the next day's fishing, set lines, and bait for other animals. But do not keep them by your camp. (Bears like fish) (see figure # P-8).

47

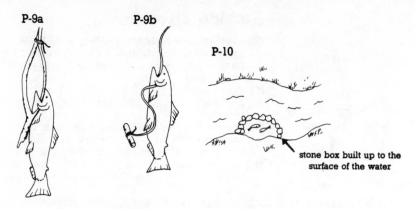

P-9a   P-9b   P-10

stone box built up to the surface of the water

* Spear fish if you can—it can be very productive.
* To transport several fish from the lake or stream improvise a stringer (see figure # P-9).
* If fishing is good you may want to make a "live" fish box. This will keep fish you have caught alive for when you may need them (see figure # P-10).
* Fish usually become more active feeders when there is a major change in the weather.
* Mussels are found in muck bottom lakes and slow moving streams. You will know they are there from their zig-zag trails in the muck. At the end of the trail you will see the tip of the mussel and can pick it out by hand. Like all shell fish, either fresh water or salt water, they should be eaten immediately and not stored without proper refrigeration.
* When you catch a fish always check in his mouth and stomach to see what he's been eating. When you find that out, start using the same item for bait, or if that isn't possible, try to imitate it.
* Make yourself up a good fishing kit, it doesn't have to be large; and keep it with you wherever you are in the wilderness.

General Methods of Fishing

Still Fishing - This is accomplished by weighting your line with lead or a rock if need be. A baited hook is attached, allowed to settle to the bottom and then the slack is taken up and the fisherman waits for a strike (see figures # P-11a & b).

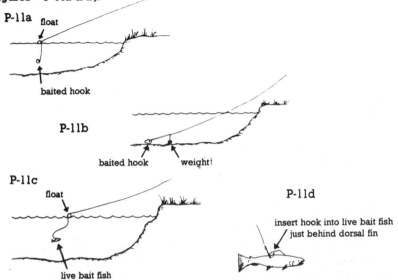

P-11a float

baited hook

P-11b

baited hook weight

P-11c

float

P-11d

insert hook into live bait fish just behind dorsal fin

live bait fish

It is a good practice to pull on your line every once in a while, then again take up the slack. This procedure may very well entice a fish to strike.

Another type of fishing is done with a lightly weighted line with a hook on the end baited with a small live chub or minnow (see figures # P-11c & d). A float is attached and cast out onto the water. The chub, if not hurt in the casting, will swim around attached to the float and attract a larger fish. You will see the float move or disappear during a strike. When fishing with large chubs for pike or lake trout, it is important to know how the predator kills and eats. He will hit the chub and kill it on his first pass then spit it out. It is important to not pull on your line yet. Wait, sometimes for over a minute, and he will be back to swallow his kill. When you see your float start to travel in one direction or completely submerge for the second time, you should count to 10 slowly and set the hook.

While still-fishing with a float for smaller fish, when the float moves it is time to set the hook.

Dry Fly Fishing - This method is used when you see fish biting the surface of a pond, lake or stream. They are feeding on airborn insects that have fallen into the water. You will want to use a tapered leader (there is one in my kit). Attach the leader to the line and the fly directly to the leader (see figure # P-12a). I have a small container of fly dope in my kits that when rubbed on the fly helps make it float. Cast the fly up stream and let it float down stream past you. Try to keep the slack out of the line and wait for the strike. When you see or feel it, instantly set the hook. If the fish are feeding and you are not getting any strikes change flies - both size and color. Naturally in the very cold fall and early spring weather when there are no airborn insects, dry fly fishing will ususally be nonproductive.

Your equipment may be limited in a survival situation and the improvised set up in figure #P-12b works well in most cases.

P-12a

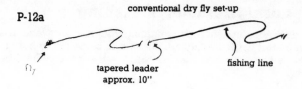

tapered leader
approx. 10''

fishing line

P-12b

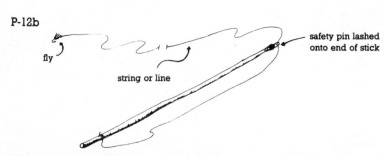

fly

safety pin lashed
onto end of stick

string or line

Spin Fishing - Spin fishing is usually done with a spinning reel which you may not have in a survival situation. What it amounts to is getting a lure out into the water and retrieving it. Spoons and spinners are ideal for this type of fishing and at times very productive. As you retrieve the lure you will want to keep it off the bottom on the way in. When you feel the strike, immediately set the hook.

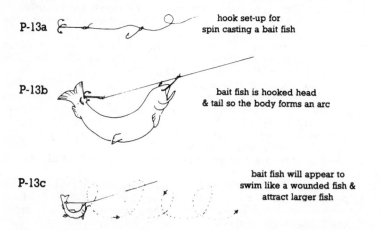

P-13a

hook set-up for
spin casting a bait fish

P-13b

bait fish is hooked head
& tail so the body forms an arc

P-13c

bait fish will appear to
swim like a wounded fish &
attract larger fish

When using this style of fishing and you have no lures available but have hooks or improvised hooks, attach a dead minnow or chub to the line as illustrated in figure # P-13a-c.

Fishing With Lead-Head Jigs - A very effective method to catch most fish, the jig, can be used alone, or with a plastic worm, or with feathers or hair attached to it (see figure # P-14a). On your retrieve you will bounce it off the bottom. Upon a strike you will set the hook immediately (see figure # P-14b).

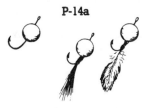

P-14a

A jig is basically a weighted hook.
Hair, feathers and bait can be added.

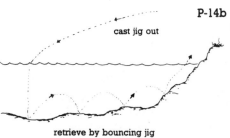

P-14b

cast jig out

retrieve by bouncing jig
along the bottom

It might be well to note here that in your travels you should be collecting pieces of hair, bird feathers, etc., to make your jigs. Also rubbing or soaking them in the decomposed fish entrails you have saved will give them the smell other fish will be attracted to.

Fishing With Spoon Type Jigs - These are especially effective when fishing through the ice. Attach the jig directly to the line and lower it to the bottom. Once you find bottom, pull it up a couple of feet and twitch it. Keep it jumping until you get a strike. Set the hook immediately.

Set-Lining - This is simply putting out a long line over night with several baited hooks attached. I like to put out two, one on the bottom and one off the bottom and I will soon find out where the fish are feeding. Check the line each morning, remove any fish and re-bait the cleaned hooks.

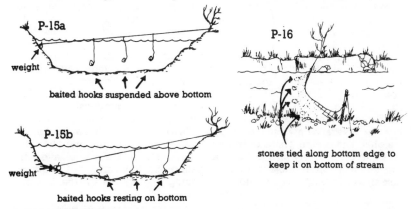

P-15a

weight

baited hooks suspended above bottom

P-15b

weight

baited hooks resting on bottom

P-16

stones tied along bottom edge to
keep it on bottom of stream

In figure # P-15 you can see two common ways of set-lining. It is wise to try both at the same time. Your bait will be the fish entrails you have been saving.

Gill-Netting - This is done by setting out a net that is constructed to catch fish by their gills as they try to swim through it. It is extremely effective to set the net up in a stream and herd the fish into it. If the stream is deep, just let them swim into it on their own accord. Pull the net in once a day and remove the fish and reset the net (see figure # P-16).

Fish Traps - These can be made from wood, stone, netting or perforated cloth. They are set in moderate depth to shallow streams and the fish are headed downstream into them (very effective). (see figure # P-6)

Spearing - Spearing is very effective when large concentrations of fish are in shallow water. Simply walk along banks or in the water, when you see a fish, spear it (see figures # P-17a-d).

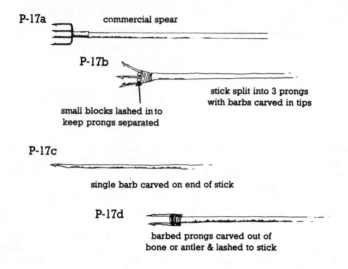

P-17a — commercial spear

P-17b — stick split into 3 prongs with barbs carved in tips

small blocks lashed in to keep prongs separated

P-17c — single barb carved on end of stick

P-17d — barbed prongs carved out of bone or antler & lashed to stick

When you are in the wilderness in a survival situation, always plan ahead in case help might be longer in coming than you think. Start collecting any items that may come in handy at a later date. With fishing materials this is also good advice. Like I mentioned before, when you come across bird feathers, animal hair, pieces of antler or bones save them. These simple items can help you assemble a vast array of tools and fishing equipment. If you are out there long enough, you may have to improvise flies, hooks, spears, fish poisons, etc. To begin with, you probably won't have a fishing rod with you so you will have to make one. You can almost always find willow growing near water and it will make an excellent fishing rod. In my kits are several safety pins, fishing line, leader material, lures, hooks, and weights. Cut a nice piece of willow about 7' long, strip its branches, and lash one of the safety pins to the smallest diameter end, and you have a fine rod that will handle most fresh-water fish, or small ocean fish. Willow will flex an astonishing amount without breaking (see figures # P-18a, b & c).

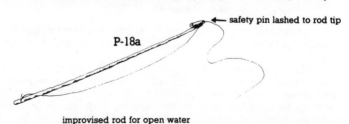

safety pin lashed to rod tip

P-18a

improvised rod for open water

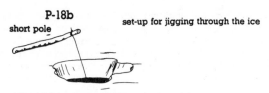

P-18b

short pole

set-up for jigging through the ice

After letting out enough line to just reach bottom,
tie off to end of pole.

Eskimo ice-fishing set-up

P-18c

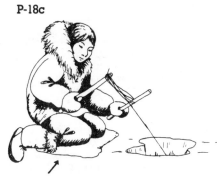

pad to keep knees from becoming wet

When a fish is hooked, it is "reeled"
in by wrapping line from one stick to another.

An improvised float or bobber can be made from a small piece of wood and if you peel off the bark it will be more easily seen. When ice fishing, the fish usually will be biting more gently and probably the finest float I've ever found is a porcupine quill. If you see a porcupine he will be your dinner but also save some quills for floats (see figures # P-19a & b).

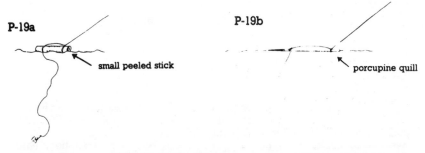

P-19a

small peeled stick

P-19b

porcupine quill

The purpose of a float is to keep your bait off the bottom, in plain sight of free-swimming fish. Also when you visually see the float being moved, you know there is a fish after your bait. It also keeps you from snagging your hook on rocks and debris found on the bottom. It's a good way to fish if the conditions are right.

Included in my kits are a few dry flies (ones that float on the surface). They are easy to lose if you are not careful and you may find yourself having to make some of your own. There are several hooks in the kit that can be fashioned into either dry or wet flies (those that are fished under the surface). This is where any feathers or animal hair you find will come in handy. Hair from deer, elk, caribou, mountain sheep, moose, and polar bear are what you want for dry flies because they are hollow and will float (see figure # P-20a). Anything will work for wet flies. They can be secured with thread from your sewing kit or clothing and with a little bit of ingenuity, you can fashion some fine flies (see figure # P-20b). As you fish them, each time you bring your fly out of the water for your next cast, snap it back and forth in the air to dry it before casting it into the water again. I like to wrap a small sliver of dry wood in the fly to aid with buoyancy. You may also want to use a slightly longer pole for fly fishing.

P-20a

dry fly

fluffed animal hair from hollow-haired
animal such as deer, moose, mountain sheep

P-20b

wet fly

← feather

← non-hollow hair
(bear, dog, human etc.)

Included in my kits are small fish spear tips. They are convenient and ready to use, but a spear can be improvised from just a piece of wood. A wood shaft and bone or antler tip is even better. A spear is an extremely effective way of procuring great numbers of fish under the right circumstances.

P-21a

wood or bone with both ends sharpened

P-21b

wood or bone or antler carved to form barb

P-21c

safety pin

← cut off

← bend pointed end

Hooks are included in various sizes in my kits but there may come a time when you must improvise. Again the bone and antler will come in handy and wood will work but has a floatation problem. Many Indians have effectively used hooks made of ivory, antler, and bone for generations (see figures # P-21a, b & c).

One problem you may encounter is not being able to get your hook and line out far enough to get into deeper water. What you should do is find a good throwing rock, wrap your line around it once, coat it with a good surface of mud and let it dry. Later you can throw the rock with the line attached far out into the water, wait a few minutes for the mud to soften and give a good tug. The line will free itself from the rock and your line will be in the deeper water. This is an old method but a good solution to the problem (see figure # P-22).

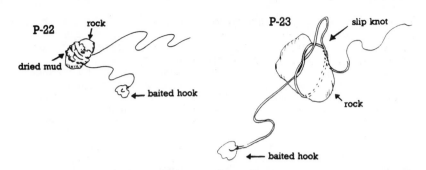

I have made some changes to this technique but most of the principles are the same. What I do is wrap my line around the rock such as to make a slip knot that will release, or hold the line fast with a thin piece of thread that will break when the line is pulled upon (see illustrations). In this way I don't have to wait for the mud to dry (see figure # P-23).

The deeper water in streams usually contains most of the fish. The reason is the subdued light, slower water, different temperatures, and a collecting place for food. When looking for deeper water in rivers or streams always look for high banks on the outside of bends. This is where the main channel of water will be and almost always the deepest area. When ice fishing it's the only place to fish and with open water it should be your first place to try.

I can't stress enough the importance of reading the water you're fishing. Just a simple eddy (place in a stream or river where the current changes, slow's down or even reverses because of the type of bend the river is taking or because of an obstacle in the water like a big rock or fallen tree) makes excellent resting, hiding and feeding holes for fish. In figure # P-24, you can see what typical steam or river might look like and how it should be read and fished.

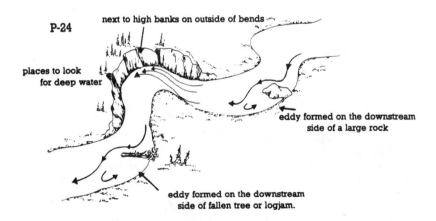

If you are landing a rather large fish, lifting him from the water to the land can present a problem because the fish becomes heavy when out of the water and you don't have the rod tip working for you anymore. You should gaff the fish while he is still in the water. He is then easily pulled out and onto land with the gaff. In each of my kits a gaff hook is included and should be fixed to a wooden pole (see figure # P-7). Don't try to hit the fish with the gaff but lay the gaff next to him and pull straight up. Large fish confined to a pool in a stream can be taken with just a gaff or spear.

In summary of this fishing chapter, remember that fish are not intelligent creatures and they always can be caught by one method or another. Their food value is unquestioned and a person could, if necessary, live entirely on fish for a prolonged period of time. In the long run you will also need some plant-type food, but fish is an excellent start. Review and memorize the "fishing tips" section. It could save your life.

And last but surely not least, learn how to read water and know where those fish are. Make the time to take the family fishing and practice what you've learned here. It can be a good education and a lot of fun for the whole family. Children love to fish and someday they may have to know how just to stay alive.

This is the fishing kit I supply in my survival kits:

Organizer Fishing Kit Box 4½" X 3" X 1¼" containing the following items:
* 4 assorted dry flies # 12 hooks
* 4 assorted dry flies # 14 hooks
* 3 large lead jigs in assorted colors # 4 hooks
* 4 small ice fishing jigs, assorted colors # 12 hooks
* 6 lead-head jigs, assorted colors # 6 hooks
* 6 short shank # 4 hooks
* 4 short shank # 14 hooks
* 4 short shank # 2 hooks
* 6 long shank # 4/0 hooks
* 1 gaff hook # 8/0 hook
* 3 swedish pimples, assorted sizes (ice fishing jigs)
* 2 large safety pins
* 1 band tied - 3-hook worm harness
* 1 Rapella lure
* 1 red & white Dare-devil
* 1 small gold spoon
* 1 small silver spoon
* 1 container of floating fly dope
* 6 4" plastic worms
* 3 2" plastic worms
* 6 3-way swivels
* 6 ball bearing snap swivels
* Assortment of lead weights
* 1 tapered fly line
* 50 yards 18# test braided nylon squidding line
* 1 steel leader - 8"
* 3 nylon leaders 20" each
* container fish poison

P-25

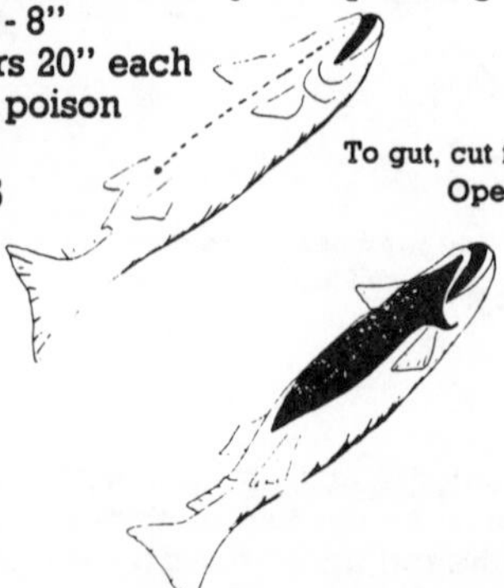

To gut, cut from anus up to inside lower jaw.
Open, remove entrails & gills.

56

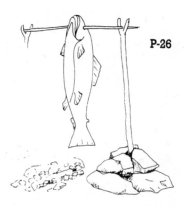

P-26

whole, gutted fish may be cooked over
hot coals by inserting a sharpened
stick through both eyes

filleting

P-27a

cut # 1

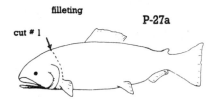

P-27b

cut # 2 - along spine

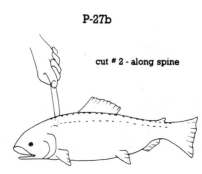

P-27c

cut # 3 - cut fillet back
away from rib cage

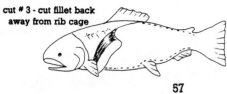

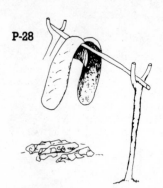

If both fillets are left attached to the tail they may easily be cooked by draping them over a pole.

P-29

Fillets will hold together better when cooked over an open fire if skins are left on.

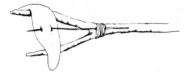

CHAPTER # 7

Food Procurement: Snares, Deadfalls & Traps

There are many ways of taking game in a survival situation. The first one we will talk about is snaring. Snaring is extremely productive and a very humane way of taking game. A snare is simply a wire or string loop placed in such a way that an animal is obliged to put its head through it. Once the snare is disturbed it will begin to tighten on the animal. When caught by the neck, which is usually the case, the animal will die quickly. Snares also have the quality of taking up very little room in your kit and naturally, weigh very little. Additional snares can be fashioned from other items in a well designed survival kit. When snares are properly prepared, handled, and placed in position they can be much more effective than a leg hold steel jaw trap.

When I'm trapping wolf or coyote which are extremely cautious animals, snares are all I use, and I might add, with deadly effectiveness. Almost all animals can be snared, from a moose to a small bird. In most survival situations this is the only way to go; it's effective, uses little energy on your part, and once set up they will be working for you even while you sleep. When we are teaching any of our longer courses we spend a considerable amount of time on the art of snaring. It is an important skill to learn and it can save your life. In the following section we will learn about the construction of snares and effective methods for setting them.

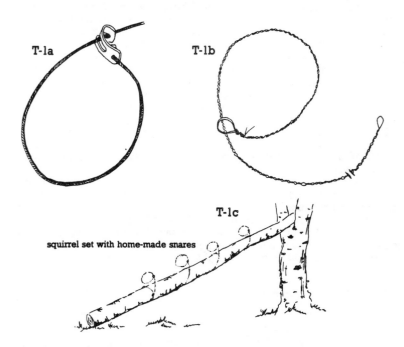

T-1a

T-1b

T-1c

squirrel set with home-made snares

In figures # T-1a & b you will see two types of snares. In figure # T-1a you see a commercial type manufactured snare with a self-locking device. This locking device allows the snare to tighten but will not let it loosen up again. It's a very effective snare.

Figure T-1b shows a home-made snare, and the one you most likely will be using in the field. It is simple to make and if designed and set properly will snap from open to a closed position with amazing speed, when just touched by the animal. I find this a strong advantage over the commercial type snares even though the latter are self locking.

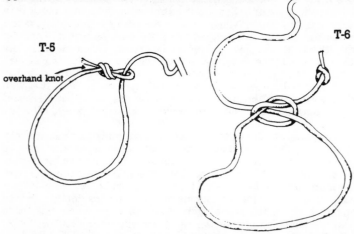

T-5

overhand knot

T-6

Figures # T-5 & T-6 show two types of string snares. Figure # T-5 shows a conventional noose that will open up if the animal backs off on the tension. In figure # T-6 is my design for a string snare. It has the unique feature of being self-locking. This is definitely a superior string snare, and I am happy to add, I have never lost an animal caught in this type snare.

Before making your snares you must consider what materials you have available for snare construction and what animal you intend to catch. In a northern survival situation your game will most likely be rabbit, snowshoe hare, and squirrel. These animals are the most plentiful and by far the easiest to catch with the exception, of course, of the unwary and simple-minded spruce grouse.

In the following examples we will be making snares for snowshoe hare. If you have assembled your survival kit properly, in it will be a good amount of snare-building material. You should have a good quality carbon wire with a gauge size of 22. You also should have either parachute cord or a similar diameter nylon cord. Again you can see the importance of nylon cord. It has helped you build your shelter, it's helped you catch fish and now it will help you snare animals.

To make the snare that is pictured in figure # T-1b you will need approximately 3' of wire. You will then fold, but don't kink, the wire in two. Place a stick next to and below the two ends. Fold the ends over the stick and wrap the wire ends around themselves tightly, at least 4 times (see figure # T-2a).

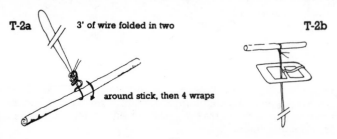

T-2a   3' of wire folded in two   T-2b

around stick, then 4 wraps

The next part makes snare making easy but is not necessary. If you have a conventional belt buckle it will work fine. Slide the wire through the opening in the buckle and bring the buckle up to the stick you have already inserted in the wire (see figure # T-2b). Next slide another stick through the loop on the other end of the wire and place it between your feet (see figure

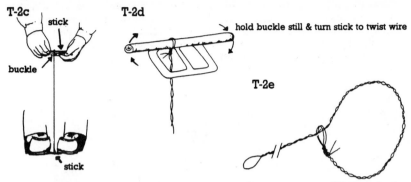

T-2c & T-2d). Place one hand under the buckle to take up the slack in the wire. With your other hand start winding the wire approximately 100 turns. Take out the sticks, slide off the buckle and assemble the snare as in figure # T-2e. Your snare is now finished. It will be perfect for snowshoe hare.

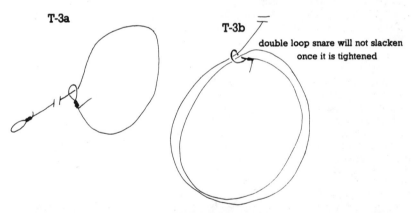

Figure # T-3 shows a similar snare made of just one strand of wire. If you are limited in wire, this might be your choice. This snare will not be as strong or as springy but if set properly will work fine.

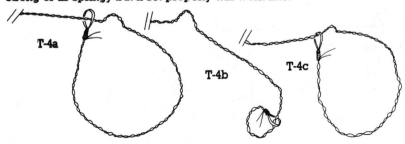

61

Figures # T-4a, b & c show how to make a proper loop and trigger. When set up right, the loop will snap from a 4" open loop to a small 2" loop, more than enough to entrap the animal. Figure # T-5 shows the conventional string snare with its fixed noose and figure # T-6 shows my style string snare with its always-tightening noose.

Now that you have decided what type of snare you are going to build and what type of animal you plan to catch, you must know how to set and position a snare to be effective. The next thing is to choose the right loop size for the animal you plan to catch. Below is a loop size chart that you can go by. It would be wise to study and remember these sizes.

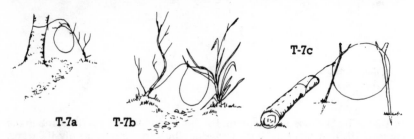

T-7a   T-7b   T-7c

The next thing you must know is the proper way to secure the loop and its distance from the ground. Figure #T-7 shows some ways of securing the loop. A wire snare is easier in this case because of it's rigidity. In any case, all you are trying to accomplish is to keep that loop open, unrestricted, so it can tighten on the animal, and keep it at the proper distance from the ground. Below are listed the proper distances of the loop to the ground for various animals.

Animal	Diameter Loop	Height Above Trail
Snowshoe Hare	4-4½"	2-3"
Red Squirrel	2½-3"	1½"
Cottontail Rabbit	3½-4"	2½"
Fox and Coyote	7-10"	10-12"
Lynx	9-10"	12"
Wolf	14-16"	16-18"
Beaver	10-12"	
Muskrat-	5"	1"

T-8a

T-8b

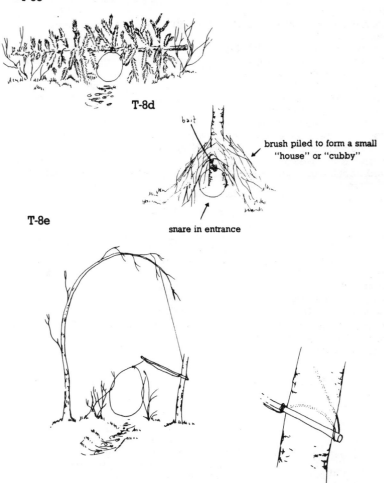

T-8d

bait

brush piled to form a small
"house" or "cubby"

T-8e

snare in entrance

Now that you know how to make and set snares you must know where to set them. This section is very important because no matter how well your snare is designed and set, it will be of no use if it is in the wrong location. If snow conditions exist it will make things easier because you can see the signs and tracks more readily and in many cases, identification becomes easier. Always snare on a heavily used trail or in an area where animals are feeding on vegetation or on a carcass, etc. If you find a den or a well-used feeding station of stored food, these are good places to set your snares.

When trapping the snowshoe hare, which will probably be your most abundant food source and the easiest to catch, remember these simple facts about this animal. First of all, like most animals, it is a creature of habit. Unless disturbed, it will do pretty much the same things each day, it will follow the same main trails and will probably sleep in the protection of a spruce forest, although it will feed on willow and alder. The trail between these two very different locations (bedding & feeding areas) will be traveled every day. When you find such a path, **DO NOT** walk in it. Stay off the path—if you destroy his easy route he may find another where your snares aren't.

Snaring in a main trail is called a trail set and is very effective for all animals.

Next, we will cover different ways of making your sets for different animals and of increasing the effectiveness of your snare and it's holding power. Some of the animals we will be talking about may not sound like your choice of meat, but if you are ever invited to a native potlatch where lynx, muskrat, beaver, etc. are served you should go. It's truly a wonderful taste treat you will never forget.

If you can build a snare so when the animal becomes caught, it will be lifted from the ground, it will be a better snare. This is not always possible, but when it is, it's a darn good idea. When an animal has all four feet on the ground, it can use its strength and maneuverability to try to free itself. Once lifted from the ground it loses this advantage and your snare becomes more effective.

In figures # T-8a - T-8e you will see how this can be easily done. I once caught, or I should say, almost caught a wolverine in fox set. He destroyed the snare and everything around it. He also walked away. At another time, again by mistake, I caught a wolverine in a marten set. The trap never would have held him except that it was a leaning pole set. The wolverine fell off and had nothing to brace his awesome power against. This shows the effectiveness of getting an animal off the ground. The marten trap would never have held the wolerine on the ground.

In the previous figures, I showed different ways of making your snare sets that will afford you the opportunity of lifting the animal from the ground. These devices are commonly called spring poles, twitch-up poles, lifting poles, snare deadfalls and toss-poles. You will also find illustrated some very effective stationary sets (those that will not lift the animal).

Things To Know And Remember

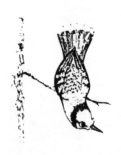

* Make sure your snares are working properly.
* Check them frequently.
* Never walk on animal trails.
* Always put out trail sets when possible.
* Whenever you can, set your snare in such a way that the animal, once caught, will be lifted from the ground.
* You should approach any captured animal that is still alive with caution.
* The entrails you saved from fishing will serve as excellent bait for almost any carnivore.
* Place brush, logs, sticks, etc. in such a manner that the animal is obliged to pass through your snares.
* Flag or mark your sets so you can find them again.

In this next section we are dealing with deadfalls. **"Deadfalls"**, like snares, were used thousands of years ago by ancient hunters for daily survival. The deadfall can be extremely effective, especially if you encounter big game in large numbers. Deadfalls are simply a heavy object (rock or log, etc.) placed in such a way that it will fall onto and kill the animal. They can be triggered in many ways and be designed for any size animal.

Probably the simplest of all deadfall methods used by our ancient hunting ancestors was to bait an animal to the base of a cliff with the hunter position-ed above. The hunter simply had to drop a heavy rock on his prey. This system was crude, and most likely resulted in many misses. It's biggest disadvantage was that without a triggering device the hunter had to stay on constant alert so as to be ready for the animal if and when it showed up. Snares are easier to build and use but if you have nothing to build a snare out of, a deadfall may be your next choice. Again you will find that nylon cord has another use and it sure makes building deadfall triggering devises much easier and versatile.

There are many types of triggers but all of these are activated either by a tripline release action, or a baited release action. A tripline release action means that the animal, while walking, will touch or trip a line, stick or pole and the deadfall device will become activated. With the baited release ac-tion the animal is attracted to the deadfall by your bait and when he pulls on it the deadfall will begin to fall. If you have found a well used trail and dead-fall building material is near-by, you will probably use a trail set activated by a tripline. If you are far from a main trail but animals are in the area you may want to build the deadfall where it's easiest and bait the animal to it. Both methods will work well; it will depend entirely on your circumstances.

In figure # D-1 you see the simple principal of the deadfall and its poten-tial if an animal is underneath. This illustration is not to be considered as an ideal set, but is meant to show you simply how most deadfalls work.

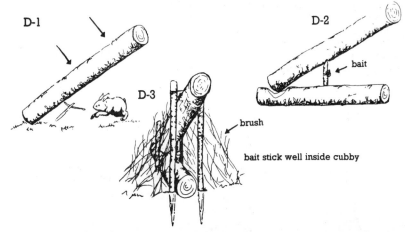

In figure # D-2 you see a set that has been improved by adding a second log called a ground log. When the fall log comes down the animal is caught between it and the ground log. There will be little or no chance of escape if the fall log is large enough. This set has a very simple triggering device which happens to be one of my favorites. Remember that usually the most reliable devices are the simplest ones. This is a baited release action trig-gering device. When the animal pulls on the bait it will dislodge the small piece of wood from the large one. The fall log will now come crashing down onto the animal which will be caught between it and the ground log.

In figure # D-3 you will see the same basic set but again improved upon. You see here that we have now added guide logs to ensure that the fall log must drop straight down onto the ground log. This principle should be ap-plied whenever possible. Also you will see that the sides of the set are obstructued with sticks and brush. This is called a cubby and the animal is obliged to enter the set from only one direction if he wants the bait. This

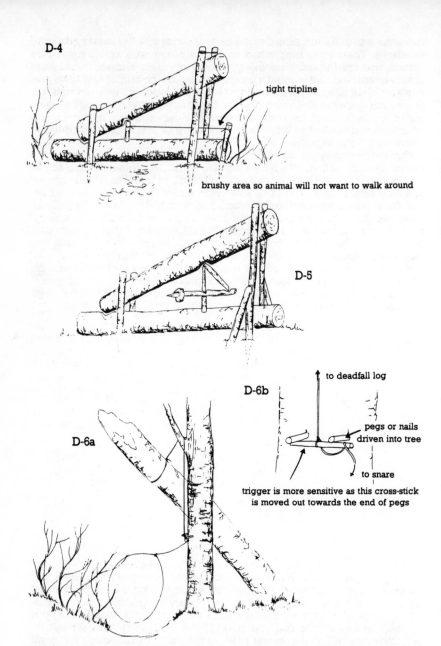

D-4

tight tripline

brushy area so animal will not want to walk around

D-5

D-6b

to deadfall log

pegs or nails
driven into tree

D-6a

to snare

trigger is more sensitive as this cross-stick
is moved out towards the end of pegs

puts the animal exactly where you want him, on top of the ground log and far into the cubby. This is a very good set and a favorite of mine. We are also using the same simple triggering device as was illustrated in figure # D-2.

In figure # D-4, a tripline release action deadfall is illustrated. As the animal passes under the fall log and is stepping over the ground log he will trip the string attached to the trigger, upsetting it and allowing the log to fall. Again we are using the same simple triggering device as before but this time without the use of bait. This would be a good trail set.

In figure # D-5 the figure 4 trigger is illustrated. It is a good trigger. I would prefer the one shown earlier but this one works well and if you have no string or cord you may have to go to this type. The figure 4 trigger takes only 3 sticks that must be strong enough to support the fall log. These sticks are notched so they will lock into one another and the weight of the fall log keeps them secure. Any disturbance will upset the trigger and it will collapse and allow the fall log to drop.

Another fine trigger for either a deadfall or deadfall drag snare combination is illustrated in figure # D-6. This type of triggering device can be easily adjusted for sensitivity. I personally like this type of trigger, but again you will need some nylon cord to fashion it.

In conclusion, remember deadfalls work; keep them and whatever device you use for a trigger simple.

SURVIVAL — TRAPPING

All small animals can also be trapped, that is captured alive in what we call a box trap, cage trap, or a tip-up slide. I prefer a properly set snare or deadfall, if for no other reason than it is a more humane way to trap. I don't like to see any animal tormented or suffering. So whenever possible I set my trapping devices to ensure a quick clean kill. If you live trap an animal you will have to be careful not to be bitten. Remember the animal will be afraid, alive and active. If by chance the animal is a carrier of rabies and you contract it, your survival experience will be horrible and extremely short.

You also will have to bring a club with you when you check your live traps. You will literally have to beat the animal to death, and there is always the chance that the animal may escape in the confusion. Again I would like to stress this is not my idea of a good humane trap, but if your situation demands it, you should have the know-how.

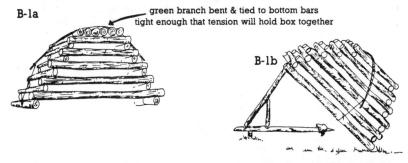

B-1a

green branch bent & tied to bottom bars
tight enough that tension will hold box together

B-1b

In figure # B-1a you can see the construction of a box trap. When the box has been built it is simply propped up on an angle by the triggering device. The animal is obliged to walk under the trap to take the bait. When the bait is moved the triggering device will be upset and the box will fall over the animal, thus confining it within the walls of the trap. In figure # B-1b the trap is set with a figure 4 triggering device. Take note that most of the trigger is outside the box so as not to prevent the trap from falling.

Figure # B-2 shows a simple cage trap. In this case the cage is stationary and a door closes behind the animal after he has entered it. You can use almost any type of triggering device you wish; I prefer the one shown. When the animal takes the bait, the trigger is upset and the cage door is allowed to close and the animal will be trapped inside. In this case the triggering device is inside the cage.

Figure # B-3 shows a tip-up slide trap. This is a very good trap and works well for almost any animal that walks or crawls on logs. It's a very simple

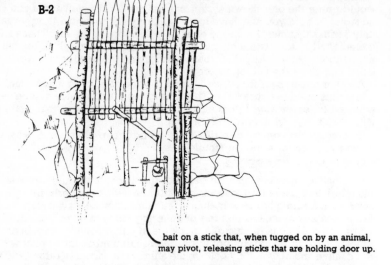

B-2

bait on a stick that, when tugged on by an animal,
may pivot, releasing sticks that are holding door up.

trap to construct and will catch even a cunning animal like a fox. This trap
can be built either from stone or wood. Stone is prefered because the
animal can't get a nail hold in the stone walls and escape. You simply build
a stone box or cylinder high enough that the animal you are after can't jump
out. Next you lay a ramp from the ground to the top of the wall that the
animal can easily climb. On the top of the wall you will balance a log and
bait it inside the trap. When the animal attempts to steal the bait he will
upset the balance of the log. Both he and the log will fall into the trap.

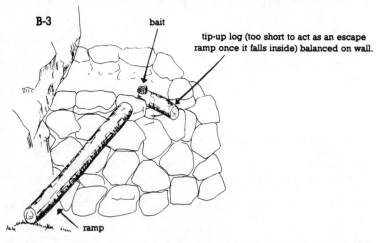

B-3

bait

tip-up log (too short to act as an escape
ramp once it falls inside) balanced on wall.

ramp

Fish can also be trapped and one method was shown in the fishing
chapter. Ocean fish can be trapped with the use of a tidal trap. Again, we
will use stone to build it. All you have to do is build a semi-circle of stone
between low and high tide mark. When the tide comes in it will carry
marine life to your trap. As the tide recedes, fish, etc. will become caught in

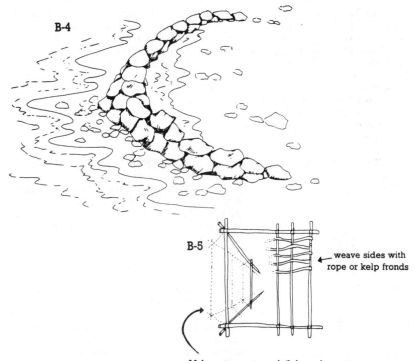

B-4

B-5

← weave sides with
rope or kelp fronds

Make entrance to crab/lobster box trap taper
inwards so animals may enter but cannot
get out.

the semi-circle. All you have to do is harvest them before the next tide or the sea gulls get at them (see figure # B-4).

Lobster and crabs can be trapped by fashioning a simple cage that will enable the creature to enter but will not allow him to get out. The trap should be set out as far as possible during low tide so it will be in deep water during high tide. Choose a rocky area and anchor the trap well to a rock or rocks. Bait the trap with the most foul-smelling rotten fish, etc. you can find along the beach and if lobster or crab are in the area you will have a tasty change of diet (see figure # B-5).

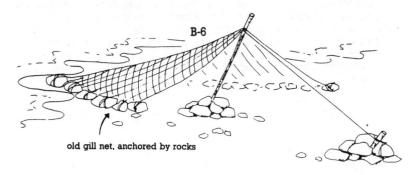

B-6

old gill net, anchored by rocks

It has been my finding that in even the most remote ocean areas the beaches are littered with debris which ranges from wood and wire to old fragmented but still useable gill nets. If you are in such an area make use of what you find. That old gill net can be set out similar to the stone tidal trap, and will catch fish. If there is a fresh water stream or river near-by that has fish in it, the net can be used again. Also wherever the tide has gone out, check the uncovered rocky areas, and tidal pools for those marine creatures like clams, mussels, oysters, etc. (These should be eaten soon, never stored. They will spoil easily). Here again is a good example of nature helping you. Nature herself has made natural traps where you can procure food (see figure # B-6).

FINAL CHAPTER TIPS, TRICKS AND THINGS TO REMEMBER

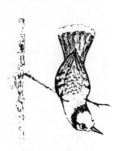

* Always disguise a trap, snare, deadfall in such a way as not to hinder its action but to break up its outline. Many animals are very clever and will recognize a trapping device if not disguised.
* Keep it simple.
* Always be on the lookout for bait for future traps.
* Never disturb or walk on animal trails you intend to use to procure food.
* When you catch an animal, dress it out immediately. If the entrails are allowed to remain in the animal for too long, especially in warm weather, the meat will begin to spoil.
* Make use of nature's natural traps.
* Approach any live animal with caution, they all can bite.
* Whenever possible set your snares, and deadfalls in well-used trails.
* Mark your sets so you will be able to find them again.
* Save all entrails and inedible scraps for future bait.
* Never store shell fish, such as clams or mussels. They should be eaten as soon as possible.
* A bent over tree used as a twitch-up will not work in very cold weather. The bent tree will freeze in position and when triggered will not be able to snap back to its original posture and lift the animal from the ground.
* When dressing out animals such as rabbits, hares & squirrels, always visually check the liver. If the animal's liver is noticeably covered with white spots, discard the animal as it may have tularemia, an infectious disease transmitted by handling the raw flesh.
* If you catch a large animal like a deer, caribou, or moose and it is below freezing, butcher the animal immediately. Once the animal has become frozen, it will be very hard to remove small sections of meat. Divide the animal into small useable portions and put them out to freeze.

CHAPTER # 8

Survival - Food Preparation and Storage

When you are in a survival situation and you come across food, you must take it then; tomorrow may be too late because that food source may be gone. If for instance when you are putting out your snares for snowshoe hare you come across a clearing and find it full of caribou, whatever you do, don't wait until tomorrow to procure that meat. Do it now. People have made that very mistake being that there are hundreds, maybe thousands of caribou as far as they can see and they will surely be there tomorrow or even next week. This kind of thinking can get you very dead. Caribou, like many animals are nomadic. They are probably just passing through and once they are gone they won't be back. If you have a rifle, now is the time to use it. If not, it's time to make some large snares or deadfalls. Watch what direction the herd in general is moving, get ahead of them and make your sets.

Once you've taken several caribou your next concern will be storage of all that meat, and that's the purpose of this chapter. If it's winter and below freezing, keeping the meat from spoiling will certainly not be a problem. During freezing conditions your main concern will be getting the skin off immediately and cutting up the meat in sections small enough that you can handle and easily cook. Always save the livers, hearts and tongues. They are very good for you and also delicious.

In fact the only animal that you wouldn't want the liver from would be a polar bear. This particular animal's liver is so rich in vitamin A that it can kill you. It should be noted here that people have gotten sick from eating the livers of sled dogs that have been primarily eating seal. The liver of any animal that is living mainly on seals should not be eaten.

Now that the meat has been divided up into small useable sections, you should build a cache. The main purpose of the cache is to keep the meat off of the ground and away from other animals. Also the cache should be covered to keep away the birds. Your cache should be built some distance from your shelter. In the winter months the bears won't be active, but in the summer, a bear in your area, or I should say you're in his area, can become a real problem. If a bear finds your cache, it's best that it doesn't happen in your camp. Figure # C-1 shows a simple cache. Note that the food is well off the ground and completely covered.

As you procure more food, such as fish through the ice, muskrat, or beaver, etc. follow the same procedure. Dress out the game, divide it into useable portions and store it in the cache. Save all the entrails in another area in a cache of their own. This is the bait you will use for future fishing, and snaring, etc. This type of winter food preservation again shows how nature is constantly working for us if we let it. Nature has supplied us with a food freezer that never breaks down, or needs repair. This is the same principle we use at our cabin in Alaska during the winter months to keep all our fish and meat that isn't canned.

If you find yourself in an extended survival situation during the summer months, nature's freezer won't be with you, but nature again has supplied you with other means to do the job. Like I've mentioned before, under no circumstances should you ever store clams, mussels or any kind of shell fish. They should be eaten right away. As you gather them, keep them out of the sun and cool. When fishing, again, keep any dead fish cool and out of the sunlight.

I prefer to keep the fish alive and then I don't have a preservation problem. The two methods I use are the live fish box we talked about earlier or

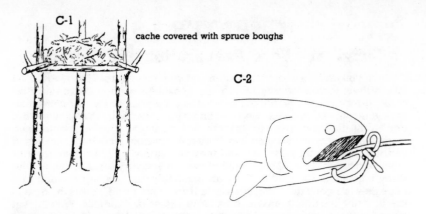

C-1

cache covered with spruce boughs

C-2

a stringer placed in the water and tied off to a solid object. When using a stringer to keep your fish alive never run it through the gills. This will in a short time kill the fish because it can not breathe. Always pass the cord through the lower jaw just behind the hard bone of the chin. This will hold the fish securely, it will be able to open and close its mouth, and its gills will be able to function as normal. Place the fish back into the water as soon as possible and tie off the other end of the stringer. This fish if not injured, can be kept alive for days. This procedure is shown in figure # C-2.

If your fish or shell fish are caught far from your camp and you will be transporting them, keep them wet, cool, and out of the sun. fish can also be stored for a day or two if you build an evaporator like the one shown in figure # C-3. Evaporation of water is a very efficient cooling process and nature supplies all the materials.

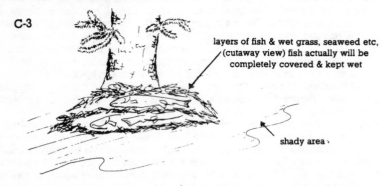

C-3

layers of fish & wet grass, seaweed etc, (cutaway view) fish actually will be completely covered & kept wet

shady area

Before going any further on the subject of food preservation, we should know some very important facts, figures, and information about fish, meat and curing. Preserving fish and red meat by brining, drying, and smoking has almost become a lost art. Each year my wife and I take in all the fish and game we will need for the year and a good share of this food is made into some of the most delicious plain and smoked sausage you have ever eaten. And just thinking of our sugar-smoked salmon is making me hungry right now. The best part is that our food is free from the chemicals and other poisons most people eat every day in food they buy at the supermarket. Home-cured food is more delicious and better for you than most store-bought food. The same curing principles can be applied in a wilderness survival situation.

The cooler you keep meat or fish, the longer it will last before spoiling. In figure # C-3 we are applying this cooling principle to keep the temperature of the fish down. As the water evaporates, it draws heat from the fish and expells it into the air, thus lowering the fish's temperature considerably. All we need to do now is to keep replacing the water lost to evaporation and we have a miniature refrigerator going. The reason why fish or meat spoils is the bacteria it contains or is exposed to. All meat and fish, whether it be fresh from the wilderness or from the supermarket shelf, contains bacteria. When we lower the temperature, most bacteria become relatively inactive, but if we allow the meat to become warm the bacteria begin to reproduce rapidly and the meat starts to spoil. Your first rule to remember is always keep raw meat or fish as cool as possible, from the time you get it until the time you eat it.

As you know, bacteria are extremely sensitive to temperature and that is exactly why a refrigerator or freezer works. On the other hand, if the temperature of the meat is raised a great amount, as in cooking, the bacteria are again disturbed. Unlike cooling and freezing where the bacteria are only made dormant or their growth slowed down, the heating process will destroy the bacteria.

All bacteria found in fish and meat are not necessarily harmful. Some of course are, with one of the most dangerous being members of the genus clostrida, particularly Clostridium botulinium, the deadly bacteria that causes food poisoning known as botulism. We would be well advised at this point to learn about this deadly microorganism. First of all, salt (sodium chloride), mixed in large enough concentration with water to form a brine will not allow Clostridium botulinum to grow. We utilize this principle each year when we bring in our salmon. We have several days without any means of refrigeration so we simply clean the fish on the spot and put them into the brine barrels. This keeps the fish from spoiling and checks the growth of Clostridium botulinum.

Keeping meat or fish cold slows the growth of Clostridium botulinum. Clostridium botulinum need a moist media in which to survive so dehydration (drying) of meat will check its growth. The organism cannot grow in a vacuum, which is why canning works.

Normal cooking temperatures will not prevent botulism poisoning once meat or fish has become spoiled by this bacteria. The thing to remember here is don't let Clostridium botulinum get started. Take care of the meat or fish right from the beginning. Keep it clean, cool and in a brine solution. If your particular survival situation puts you in a salt water area your brine is already started for you. Most beaches are loaded with well-washed debris. Find a metal container, fill it with salt water and start a fire under it. As the water boils and evaporates, keep adding more salt water. By doing this you are increasing the amount of salt in the container. Finally, fill the container

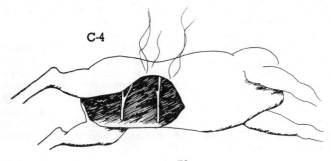

C-4

to the top and let it cool. You now have a suitable brine for later use. Sea water is not salty enough to be sterile. To make a bacteria killing brine, you must concentrate the salt by evaporation and sterilize it by boiling.

Some meats can contain trichinae which is the organism that causes trichinosis. This internal parasite is very sensitive to temperature and dies when its temperature is raised to 138 degrees F. Cook all your meat well and this and most other parasites and microorganisms will be killed.

You can see now why it is so important, to immediately after taking a fish or animal, remove its entrails and start the cooling process. With big game such as deer or moose, you need to prop the cavity open immediately after gutting to get that heat out (see figure # C-4). As you know, bacteria needs a moist media to live in. Knowing these facts, let's go through a step by step example of taking care of a deer we just snared or shot in a survival situation far out in the bush during the summer.

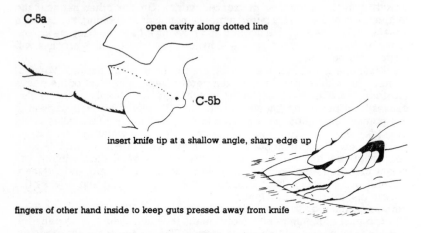

C-5a

open cavity along dotted line

C-5b

insert knife tip at a shallow angle, sharp edge up

fingers of other hand inside to keep guts pressed away from knife

Our first step upon approaching the animal is to make sure it is dead. If the animal's eyes are open but not moving, the animal is probably dead. Make sure by nudging the animal from a distance with a stick or similar prod. Once we are sure the animal is dead we will immediately open the animal up with a knife, (see figure # C-5) being careful not to stick the knife in too far and puncture the internal organs. Now we roll the animal onto its side and pull out all the internal organs, being sure to also remove all of the lungs.

At this time we will separate out the liver and heart to start them cooling. If we decide to move the entire animal to a more suitable location to butcher it, we will prop open the gut and chest cavity with sticks to help the animal cool down as quickly as possible, but leave the skin on until we have moved the carcass to where we plan to butcher. The next step is the removal of the skin. When skinning the animal be careful not to rub the hair side on the meat or you will be adding bacteria to your meat.

Once the skin has been removed the carcass should be quartered (see figure # C-6). In contrast to the winter procedure, we will not cut the meat into sections. The reason for this being the more surface area we expose to the air, the greater the chance of contamination from airborne bacteria. We now take the quarters, rib section, and neck and hang them in a cool area away from the sun. The air will immediately start to dry the outside of all the pieces and a hard bacteria-resistant crust will be formed. As you can see, the air that carries bacteria can also help us guard against it. Nature again is there to help us if we let it.

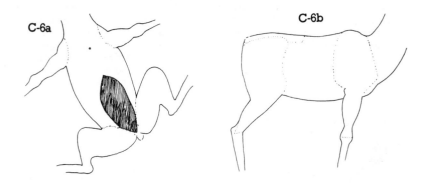

C-6a

C-6b

Next, don't forget to remove that tongue; it will make a good meal. At this point I would start several small smokey fires, not close enough to heat the meat, but to envelope it in a good hard wood smoke. Never use a conifer to smoke meat, it will ruin the flavor. The reason that we are going through this smoking process is to keep away flies and other insects while the meat is crusting over. We know that insects do not like smoke and they will not like the smokey flavor on the outside of the meat. If the meat is kept cool and dry it can be held in this condition for a long period of time.

My next move would be to make a nice cooking fire and enjoy that liver. And tomorrow we eat steak. Liver is not only the most nutritious part of the animal, but the one that will spoil quickest. The meat should be stored in your covered cache and away from your camp. It's summer now and the bears are on the move. If I felt my food supply was threatened by a bear I would certainly build a deadfall at the cache. When attempting to kill a bear, especially a large grizzly, you will need as heavy a fall log as you can lift, and then add as much extra weight as you can to it. Bears should never be underestimated. They are smart, built like a tank, and extremely strong! See figure # C-7 for deadfall details.

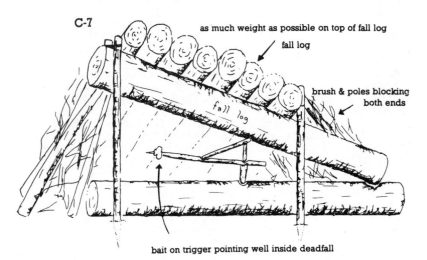

C-7

as much weight as possible on top of fall log

fall log

brush & poles blocking both ends

fall log

bait on trigger pointing well inside deadfall

75

Even with all the precautions we've exercised so far the meat will eventually spoil if not consumed in a reasonable amount of time. I would certainly take a portion of the meat and dry smoke it. As we already know, the bacteria we are concerned with needs a moist media to live on. By dry smoking we will be removing almost all the moisture, thereby giving the bacteria no place to live. We will at one point raise the temperature of the meat to over 138 degrees, and we will add hardwood smoke to it. The end product is meat bacteria do not want to live in, and insects won't like.

C-8

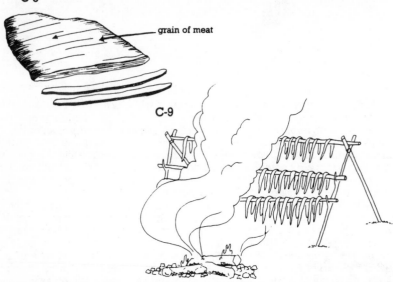

grain of meat

C-9

We will start by taking some of the meat and cutting it in long thin strips with the grain (see figure # C-8). We will then make a drying rack and start the dehydration process. This can be done with a fire or good strong sunlight. At the same time, have a nice smokey hardwood fire going (see figure # C-9). When the meat seems almost dry move it closer to the fire for a few minutes to raise the temperature. When your strips of meat are hot to the touch, move them back away from the fire and continue to dry until they become brittle. If kept in this condition the meat will last a very long time. You can chew on it like jerky or cook it in water to re-hydrate it.

A very common misconception is that smoking cures meat. Smoking does not cure meat; it merely adds flavor and discourages insects. It has absoulutely no affect on bacterial growth. What does have a devasting effect on bacteria is dehydration, very cool or very hot temperatures, and salt. If you can make a brine and soak the meat strips in it before the dry-smoking process, it's even better. I might add here that sugar is also a preservative and can be used like salt, remembering that sugar is not quite as effective as salt.

CHAPTER # 9
Water Procurement

In this chapter you will learn how to find, collect, and even generate water. I can not stress too much the importance of water to you in a survival situation. A person can go for weeks without food, but go just a few days without water and you are in big trouble. You know that two of the main killers in the wilderness are panic and hypothermia, but just as deadly is dehydration, and in many cases dehydration can and will lead you to hypothermia and panic. There has been a great deal of research done on this subject in the last few years, and I might add, with some startling results. Remember always that anytime you are lost or stranded in the wilderness, water procurement is of the utmost importance. I only have one definition of dehydration and that is dehyration is a killer.

Let us start with some facts and information about your body and its water requirements. Let's find out exactly what happens to your body when it requirements for water are not met.

The food we ingest each day contains anywhere from one to two quarts of water. Each day we also drink, in one way or another, 1½ to 2 quarts. During the oxidation process of metabolism our bodies form another half a quart of water. You can see here that normal daily, low stress conditions our bodies are receiving from 2 to 4 quarts.

We lose each day through urine, expired air, and insensible perspiration approximately 2 to 3 quarts. During time of heavy breathing or obvious sweating your fluid loss will be a great deal more. When working in high or very low environmentsl temperatures, an alarmingly great amount of fluid can be lost. This loss alone can take from 2 to 5 quarts of water from your body per day. When adding this figure to your normal losses of 2 to 3 quarts, you can see it is very possible to lose and have to replace up to 8 quarts of water per day.

Remember, however much water your body loses you must replace all of it. If you do not replace all of it, dehydration has begun. The most important organ in your body, your brain, will start to malfunction. The symptoms will be similar to exhaustion, or hypothermia, i.e., lessened awareness of your surroundings, slowed reflexes, decreased coordination, and difficulty making rational decisions. A person suffering from this condition always tends to do things the easy way rather than the right way, or will neglect essential tasks all together. As you can see, this is an extremely serious situation and technically a form of shock, just as is serious bleeding from a wound. Once your decision making is impaired, mistakes become more frequent and more serious and this situation can lead only to death.

Another usually overlooked but extremely important part of this dehydration business is understanding the electrolyte balance of your body. Both urine and sweat contain a good deal of salt and electrolytes. When these are lost along with water through urination, sweating, and especially vomiting and diarrhea, they need to be replaced. Otherwise what will happen at this point is even though you are replacing the water that you lost, your body will try to expel it in order to maintain important electrolyte balance. What must be replaced is primarily sodium chloride (salt), potassium, and calcium.

Ideally you should at this point have salt or salt tablets and be eating well-balanced meals. In a survival situation this may not be possible. For this reason it's a good idea to always carry some salt tablets in your survival kit. As you can see, they could save your life. Assuming that you are in less than ideal conditions - you have no salt or salt tablets, and your diet is less than well-balanced, you will have to use what nature provides.

If available, any form of edible fruits or berries will provide some electrolytes. If you have access to sea water it should be boiled and ½ to 2 cups drunk per day. Let your body cravings dictate the amount - it will usually be right. Also, if you're on the seashore, kelp (see plant chapter) is an excellent source of salts and electrolytes. There are significant amounts of salt and electrolytes in all meat and fish especially salt water fish and shell fish. If you don't have access to meat yet, instead of drinking plain water, make tea from the plants listed in the plant chapter. If you have access to a very limited amount of meat be sure to cook and eat all the blood; this is rich in salt and electrolytes.

Always remember dehydration is a serious killer that attacks your brain.

We will now talk about actual water procurement in the wilderness. In the winter time when snow and ice are available, water procurement can become an easy job. However, you should never attempt to eat snow or ice. The calories consumed in the process far outweigh the benefit of the small amount of water gained. If you were very thirsty and began to eat snow, before the thirst could be satisfied you would be starting into hypothermia.

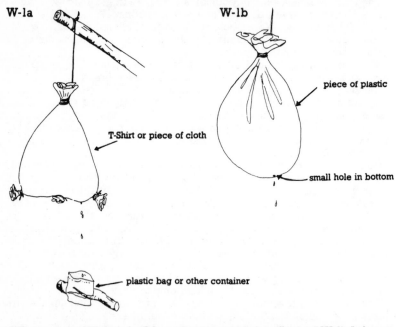

W-1a

W-1b

T-Shirt or piece of cloth

piece of plastic

small hole in bottom

plastic bag or other container

What you should do is build a water generator (see figure # W-1). I always keep an already made up water generator in my parka so if I need it, it's there. You, if necessary, can improvise one from your T-shirt or any piece of cloth. Tie the neck and arms of the T-shirt closed and fill it with snow, constantly banging it on the ground to compact the snow (make it more dense). Hang the bag near your fire and wait. In about ½ hour or so the generator will start to drip from one spot. Place any kind of collector under this drip and your water problems are over.

Never let the generator completely run out of snow; keep adding more snow when necessary. Once started this type and size generator will supply more than enough water for 2 people's needs. This is an excellent way to procure drinking water in the winter. Just be careful not to get the water generator too close to the fire. You won't want to burn a hole in what might be the only spare piece of cloth you have.

If you have a cooking container and you choose to melt snow or ice in it over a fire, that's fine also. When using this method and you have the choice of ice or snow, use the ice. You will get more water from a pan full of ice than you would a pan of snow. The ice is more dense and naturally will yield more water. When using this method to make water, be careful not to burn the bottom of the pan when first starting the melting process. Once the bottom is covered with water you'll be safe to use more heat.

If your survival situation puts you on sea ice, the older sea ice will have lost most of its salt content. This old ice will probably become your source of drinking water. The old ice will have rounded corners, and have a blue tint. Any sea ice that is milky gray in color is what is called new sea ice and will contain far too much salt to drink. Snow may have been soaked by the open ocean spray. This snow is not suitable to melt and drink. You'll have to look in another spot for fresh snow.

In the winter my choice is usually to start a water generator going. This method leaves me free to perform other important tasks while the water is being made. In winter, whenever possible, drink warm water. It helps you guard against hypothermia.

Summer water procurement is different. Naturally when you set up your permanent camp, you should choose a location close to a fresh water supply if possible: a river, a lake, a pond, or even a small creek. In the north country we are blessed with an abundance of the above mentioned water sources that man hasn't figured out how to pollute yet, so whenever possible try to camp near a good water source. If for whatever reason you can't find an open water source, don't panic; you are still going to be O.K. There is water nearby, you just can't see it yet. The first thing to do is use your eyes and look around. Take a little walk and survey the whole area with your eyes, and at the same time keep your ears open and listen for water. Because of the peace and quiet the wilderness affords, you will be able to hear things that you normally wouldn't.

A good example of this is the time when Gretchen and I were in an unfamiliar area and looking for a good place to make camp. Water was naturally one of our first concerns but there was no sign of it in our area so we spread out and started on what we call a look-and-listen walk. We walked slowly and quietly, noticing everything from the tiny world of lichens beneath our feet to the birds in the sky, every once in a while stopping, closing our eyes and listening to what could be heard. This method has been extremely effective for us and during this particular expedition it proved effective again.

Within about an hour Gretchen signaled me to come in her direction. I did and she motioned for me to listen. Sure enough, the sound of water splashing on a rock could be heard. We walked quite a ways before finding the origin of the sound but when we got there it was worth it. It was a miniature water fall coming from the side of a very rocky mountain. We naturally made camp there, drank a lot of water, and slept a peaceful sleep in another wonderland of beauty. The thing I would like you to remember here is that even though it may seem water is no where to be found it may be very close by if you look and listen.

Another time when there seemed to be no obvious sign of water we saw two mallard ducks fly overhead, circle some distance away, set their wings, and go down, disappearing through the trees. That naturally was our answer. Mallards and all ducks like water and when they land it is usually on or near water. We walked in that direction and found a beautiful small hidden lake. We never would have walked in that direction if we hadn't seen the ducks.

Again, I would like to stress, the importance of looking and listening. I've had students ask me what am I looking and listening for during these walks. My answer can only be "How the heck do I know?" Listen and look for everything. If you can learn to do this you will find yourself in a new and special world, and experience a special closeness with what is around you.

W-2

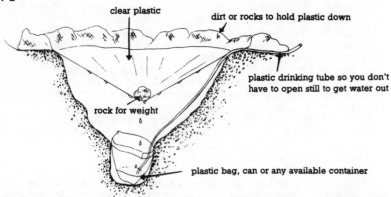

clear plastic

dirt or rocks to hold plastic down

plastic drinking tube so you don't have to open still to get water out

rock for weight

plastic bag, can or any available container

There may be circumstances where water procurement may become more of a task. Let's take a look at what can be done in these cases. A solar still can be made and works well. You will need a piece of plastic that should be in your survival kit and something to collect water in. In figure # W-2 you can see the construction of a solar generator or still. You will want to dig your hole where the heaviest concentration of underground moisture will be. Some good examples can be seen in figure # W-3a, # W-3b, and # W-3c.

W-3a

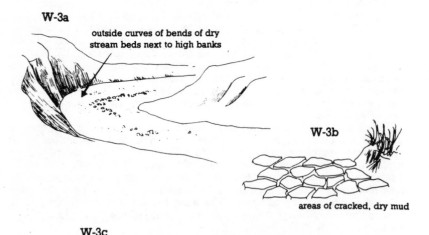

outside curves of bends of dry stream beds next to high banks

W-3b

areas of cracked, dry mud

W-3c

low or spongy areas with heavier vegetation than surroundings

A solar generator or still will not only collect water, it will purify it. This type of generator will even distill pure water from urine, draw moisture from poisonous plants, etc., or purify a very polluted water source. Figure # W-4 shows collected polluted water being purified and recollected.

W-4a

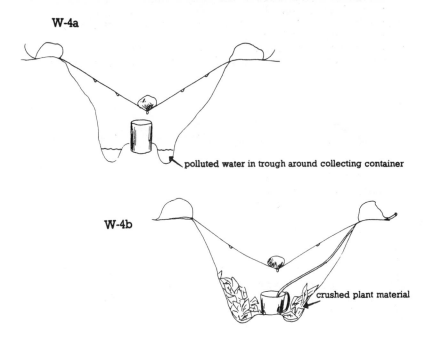

← polluted water in trough around collecting container

W-4b

crushed plant material →

The following tips and tricks and general rules have been tested and used probably ever since there was man. All of them can help you find water, or make impure water safe to drink.

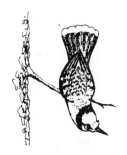

* Do not drink sea water. It contains too much salt. (A little, as explained earlier in the chapter can be used to readjust your body's electrolyte balance.)
* Whenever possible purify water before you drink it.
* In the northern latitudes, melted snow ice, and rainwater (collected directly) as a general rule can be considered drinkable without purification.
* Water that is clear and runs a long way through gravel can usually be considered more pure than stagnent or water running over mud.
* Boiling water is probably the best simple means of water purification.
* The general rule for boiling water to promote purification is boil for at least two minutes (add an additional minute for each one-thousand feet of altitude).
* Water is completely purified when collected from a solar still.
* Never melt ice or snow in your mouth.
* After a rain, fresh clean water can be found in depressions of rocks and leaves of plants. (see figure # W-5 for collection).
* Dried up river beds can be a good source of water. (see # W-3a).

* Low lands and valleys are good places to look for surface water or streams.
* Water will find its way directly out of mountains especially in rocky areas (this type of water is usually very pure).
* Very cold water is usually more pure than warm water.
* Look for abnormally lush growth of plant life (they are getting a lot of water from somewhere) (see figure # W-6 seep hole).
* There is drinkable surface water all over the tundra areas.
* Sea water can be converted to fresh water by distilling (see figure # W-4)

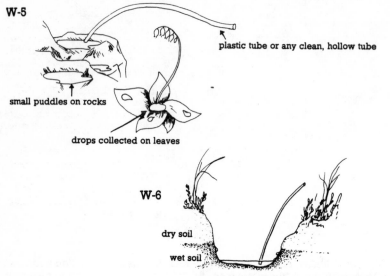

W-5

plastic tube or any clean, hollow tube

small puddles on rocks

drops collected on leaves

W-6

dry soil

wet soil

dig several inches below level of wet soil,
wait for water to seep into hole & drink through a tube

CHAPTER # 10

Signaling

This chapter deals with different types of signaling techniques. We will cover both commercial and improved signals and discuss their applications and usefulness. Proper signaling can make the difference between being located or not. A properly made signal can and will be seen from several air miles away and a poor signal may never be seen. Like anything else, there is good and poor signaling equipment on the market. You must be careful in what you buy and I truly hope this chapter can help you save money and maybe your life.

In most cases if you are missed the search and rescue team will probably be searching from the air with small planes. A good lesson to remember here is whenever going in the wilderness or flying over it, tell someone your planned route. If you don't make it to your destination someone will know that something is wrong and also will have some idea where to at least start a search. Another fact to remember is that when down in the wilderness the search planes will be flying during the day and not at night. Night signaling in most cases is useless because the most productive searching can be done during the daylight hours. In some extreme cases night search will become necessary but this is the exception and not the rule. Knowing this we will stress mostly day light signals. Also knowing that a search and rescue team will most likely searching from the air we will have to put ourselves in the searchers' seat and constantly be wondering what our signal will look like from the air and not from the ground. Because of this we will be covering mostly ground to air signaling geared generally for daytime use. We will however cover other aspects and methods of signaling.

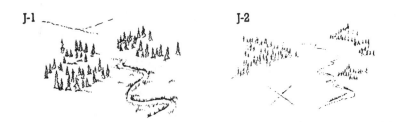

J-1   J-2

Let us begin with what makes signals work or not work. One of the major facts about signaling in the wilderness is that there are very few straight unbroken lines. In figure # J-1 you can see what I'm talking about. This is a typical areial view of a section of the subarctic wilderness. As you can see from the figure, there are no continuous straight lines and this is what the rescue pilot is used to seeing. In figure # J-2 you see the same view but this time there is a signal made from spruce boughs. Notice now the straight lines of the signal stand out. This is a good signal and it has been improvised completely from the wild, during the summer season.

This signal also tells the pilot a story and has a definite meaning. It is one of the standard accepted distress signals found in the reference section. This signal means "unable to proceed". This signal has served its purpose: Number one, it attracted the attention of the search plane pilot, and number two it has given the pilot your message. Another reason why the signal stands out is the color contrast between it and what it is built on. Its size is also big enough not to be missed. In figure # J-3 notice the actual ground dimensions of this signal. This is very important because what looks large on the ground may not be noticed from the air. These are the accepted measurements for both military and civilian rescue personnel.

J-3   J-4

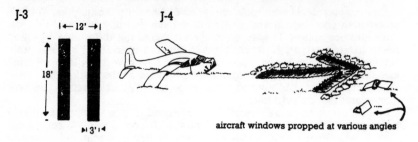

aircraft windows propped at various angles

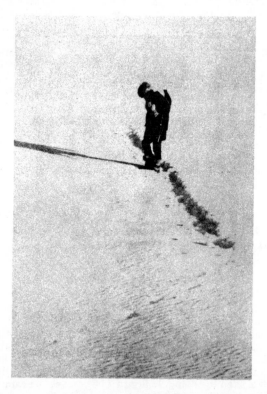

If you are down in an aircraft, the aircraft itself becomes a fine signal so long as it is in open country. If you choose to leave the aircraft and set up camp some distance away, leave a signal so the pilot can find you (see figure # J-4). This signal is well known and means "am prceeding in this direction". This signal is built by removing the muskeg from the area to expose the soil; again, a color contrast with straight lines. Also notice how the aircraft stands out and some windows have been removed and placed at better angles. The windows can reflect the sun's light like mirrors.

The finest ground to air signal you can use, short of a forest fire, is a good smoke signal. If applicable to your situation it should be used. A good smoke signal positively cannot be missed during the day from the air. Engine oil will burn smokey black and the addition of the aircraft tires will make it even better. Let the air out first then cut off the valve stem. This will keep the tire from exploding when burned (see figure # J-5).

When no outside materials are available, you can still make a fine effective smoke signal that can be seen for miles. The secret with these signals is they have to be ready when a plane is spotted so that all you have to do is light them. You will not have the time to gather materials then.

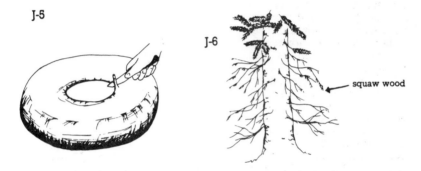

J-5

J-6

← squaw wood

As soon as you can after the initial accident, after you attend to any medical problems, gather your smoke signaling materials and set them up. Make sure your matches, flint and steel, or other fire igniting device is ready. Get your initial fire completely ready to go. Have your green spruce boughs near-by in a pile or piles. One of the most common mistakes people make is not having enough green spruce boughs to completely cover and smother the fire when they are ready. For this type of signal you will collect a huge pile of squaw wood (the dead lower branches if the spruce tree) this pile should be at least 6' x6'x 6' (see figure # J-6). Build this pile on your incline poles and start gathering your green spruce boughs. You will need a pile at least as big as the squaw wood pile and have it piled only a few feet away. Next, set your small tinder and fire starter under the squaw wood pile (see figure # J-7).

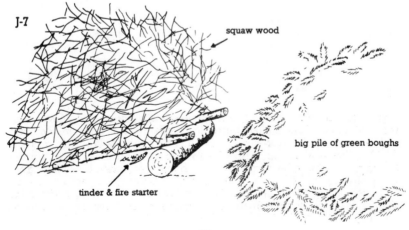

J-7

squaw wood →

big pile of green boughs

tinder & fire starter

You are now ready for any airplane at any time. When you see a plane, start your tinder, add fine squaw wood. Within seconds, you will have a huge fire. When it's at its peak, start throwing the green spruce boughs on and completely smother the fire (see figure # J-8). At this point huge billows of thick white smoke will arise that cannot be missed. I would set up several of these fires and light them one by one to create as much smoke as I possibly could. This is the finest daytime signal you could possibly hope to have and it will attract attention from a long ways away.

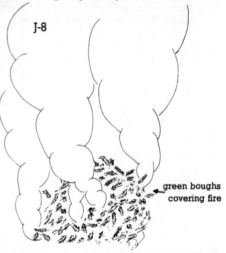

If you have an orange smoke signal in your kit, this would be the time to use it. Place it near the base of the fire and the smoke signal will begin to turn orange in color. This procedure adds to what you already have, but is not necessary.

Another excellent ground to air signal which can be used alone or with other signals is a piece of florescent orange cloth like I always carry with me in the bush. Your large survival kit should have one (see figure # J-9). This signal placed in the open can be seen for miles. When the sun is shining on it becomes so bright it's hard to look at. Here we are using color contrast to do our signaling job.

J-8

green boughs covering fire

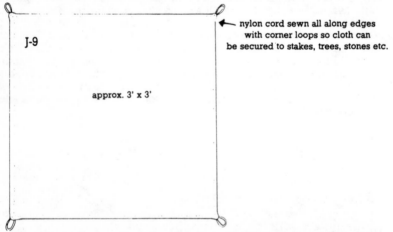

J-9

nylon cord sewn all along edges with corner loops so cloth can be secured to stakes, trees, stones etc.

approx. 3' x 3'

The signal mirror can be a fine day-time signaling device whenever there is bright sunlight. The military mirror is excellent and so are some commercial versions. The mirror should have a see-through hole in the center in which a "fire ball" is captured. When you aim this "fire ball" at an aircraft, the mirror will be at the correct angle to signal the aircraft. If you just have a plain mirror you can use your fingers to sight the mirror directly on the aircraft (see figure # J-10). A signal such as this can be seen for many miles. Your survival kit should contain one of these mirrors. They are inexpensive and they work.

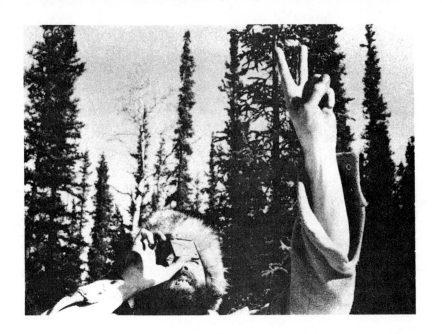

J-10

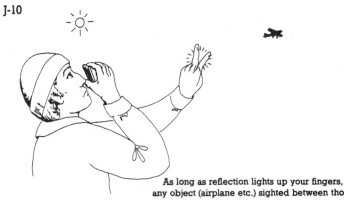

As long as reflection lights up your fingers,
any object (airplane etc.) sighted between those
fingers will be in the path of the flash from your mirror.

While we are talking about commercial signaling devices, flares should be mentioned. Flares are made to produce light. Some produce white light and some produce a red light. Both are very visible at night and both are poor during the day, the white light being the worst. Flares come in hand-held and aerial models. Aerial flares are designed to make either a white or red light, and at night are rather impressive. But during the day I would build a smoke signal and have a better chance of being rescued. If you have the room, flares are a good idea for your kit, but certainly not a necessity.

A good winter signal for when no materials other than snow can be found is shown in figure #J-11. This is called a snow-block-shadow signal. By digging out snow blocks, stacking them using the straight line principle, you

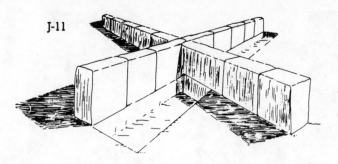

J-11

set blocks up next to the trench you
dug them out of for additional depth

will be able to create a strong shadow as long as there is sun. This signal is
hard to see from the ground level but excellent from the air.

Another good winter signal is the placing of spruce boughs on the
borders of an area you have snowshoed down (see figure # J-12). This signal
gives good contrast and in figure # J-13 you can see another variation.

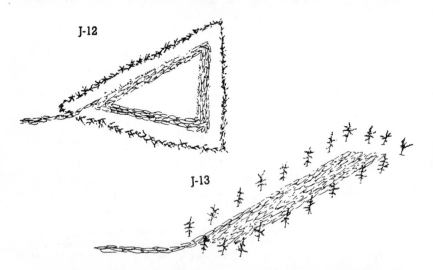

J-12

J-13

A good bright fire is probably one of the best night signals you could
have and if it fits your situation you should use it. A whistle will carry further
and last longer than your voice. They are inexpensive and good to have in
you kit. If you spot another person, that whistle may come in handy. The
reason it is so effective is its shrill pitch which will sometimes carry over
loud background noises such as a water fall even better that a gunshot.

Another excellent and very inexpensive signalling device is a survival
blanket, sometimes called a space blanket. What is nice about it is that it fits
in a shirt pocket when folded and when opened it measures a full 56" x 84".
It weighs almost nothing. These space blankets can have many uses and for
signaling they are great. In figure # J-14 you can see two excellent signals
made from these blankets. Little pieces of this blanket hung from a string

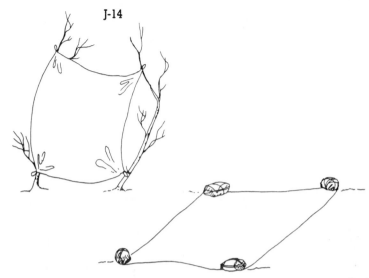

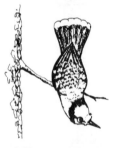

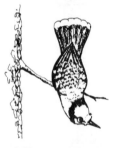

will also attract curious animals directly to your snare, or deadfall. This is a signal to an animal to investigate something new. I use this trick on my regular trapline each year and it's very effective.

RULES AND TRICKS TO REMEMBER ABOUT SIGNALING

* Always set your signals out as soon as possible. That airplane may be just minutes away.
* A good signal can be seen a long ways from the air.
* A good signal has a lot of color contrast with its surroundings.
* A good signal is made up of straight lines (unless smoke or fire is used).
* The best daytime signal is smoke.
* The best nighttime signal is fire (light).
* If necessary, use materials from your downed aircraft to make a signal, (fuel, oil, tires, and the aircraft itself).
* Make your signal as large as possible.
* Always think what your signal will look like from the air.
* Take advantage of anything you may have that is reflective (space blanket, window glass, mirror, etc.).
* Always place your signals in the open where they can be seen.
* Improvise with what you have at hand.

I would like to end this chapter with a true life anecdote that happened a few years ago to an Alaskan pilot. It is an excellent example of signaling and how quick-thinking and improvisation saved another life. The pilot's plane crashed into a very large, cold and deep lake. The pilot managed to get on top of his plane but it was slowly sinking. A tin can floated up from within the aircraft. Almost at the same time he saw another float plane in the distance. He recovered the shiney tin can and used it as a mirror to signal the approaching plane. The other aircraft did see the flashing signal and rescued the first pilot before his plane completely sank. Without that signal the other plane would have kept going without knowing of the emergency.

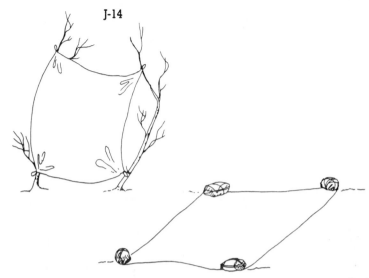

CHAPTER # 11
Walking Out

If you decide to walk out, the whole business of wilderness survival will take on a new dimension. In this chapter I will talk about and explain the tricks and techniques I use. But remember, unless you really have your survival skills down pat I would again have to advise you against it. To start with let's make a list of the most important things you are going to encounter and have to deal with.

* When walking out and on the move you will have no permanent signals already set up ahead of you to notify an aircraft where you are. We will cover this in depth in this chapter and this is a very important issue.

* You can only take with you what you can easily carry. This means little food and water.

* You must be able to walk in a fairly straight line - (that is, on one straight predetermined bearing).

* You will be burning a tremendous amount of calories by walking and giving up more water than normal, (both the water and calories must be replaced each day).

* You will have to make a new camp each evening.

* You will have to be very cautious in choosing your route to avoid dangerous terrain.

Let's take the list and look into these potential problems. First of all, signaling is very important if you plan to be rescued. Your first move before leaving camp should be to set up some sort of permanent signal (see figure # H-1). If it is winter and it snows after you've left but before a search plane arrives, your signal will probably be covered or camouflaged with snow. The purpose of your signal is to let the search aircraft know you are in the area, have left, and what direction you took.

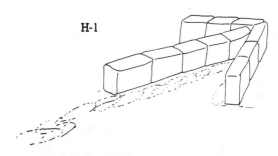

H-1

The only signal that I know of that will give you a half chance under unattended snowy conditions is the snow-block-shadow signal, if drifting isn't too bad. Your signal should be built as large as possible in an open area and pointing exactly in the direction you intend to travel. Do not clutter the area around the signal with a lot of your tracks. Walk in and out of the signal area in the same set of tracks. It is also a good idea along the way as you find suitable open areas to build similar signals so you can be followed.

If you have a signal mirror, have it in a good spot ready to use if you see an aircraft. The same goes for a flare or any other signaling device you may have.

As you know, the best daytime signal you can have is smoke but you won't be walking out with a pocket full of smoke ready to release at any time. You can however, have a pocket full of fire starting material and enough light dry squaw wood tied on your back so as to be able to start a signal fire in minutes if you are in the right terrain. This trick could save your life. If you are in an area where there is more squaw wood and green spruce boughs, you will probably be able to signal the aircraft in time. The fire starting materials you have in your pocket and the squaw wood on your back will get that fire going, as you RUN and gather the rest. This will give you an edge on time and in this case, time is so important.

If there is no snow, your signal can be made of spruce boughs or even stone if placed in the proper area (see signaling chapter).

When you leave, you must take with you your most important tools, and a closed water container if you have one. If you have dried meat and fish, they will be light and you should take only what you can easily carry. If you have a weapon of any sort, have it ready for use as you walk. You will have to take game when you see it. When you come across edible plants and berries, eat some while enroute and save some for your evening meal. Be constantly searching for water and drink as much as you can when you find it. If you have a water container, fill it whenever you can.

When you make camp for the night, always set out as many snares as you can. In this situation you need every edge you can get. And if you come across water that may have fish in it, take the time to fish it. I might add here, if the fishing is good take several more than you can eat and dry them before you continue on your way. The next leg of your journey may produce little food. Remember your walking is burning calories that you must replace. And while you walk, try not to rush and start sweating. You don't want to give up any more water than you have to. Remember, this mistake alone could kill you.

As you walk out, you must be conscious of walking in a straight line. The chapter on direction-finding has the information you will need here.

When you make camp each evening it should do the job but be simple. Always allow enough time to make camp while you still have light. Always keep your tools and equipment organized, and inventory them each day; you can't afford to lose anything.

As you choose each day's route, exercise caution. You will not want to walk through a swampy or boggy area. It's dangerous and you will get wet and cold. If you ever are walking in a low-land area and it feels as though the ground under your feet is unstable, you may be walking on a quaking bog. This is a body of water that has a layer of vegetation covering its surface. You can easily punch through the surface cover and drown. When you see these swampy, boggy or unstable areas, go around them, never through them.

When you make your plan to go a certain way and it turns out to be more than you bargained for, don't chance it. This is how injuries and deaths happen. Know your limitations and act accordingly. Those who venture in the real rugged wilderness are like bush pilots: there are old ones and bold ones but there are no old, bold ones. This is a good little jingle to always remember. The people that want to act macho and exceed their limitations should stay in the city where they can get away with it. The wilderness will kill them. For example, let's say you are in the mountains and the area you planned to go through has an impassable area in it. If you skirt just below it instead of re-routing you will have to cross a hundred yards of scree (a loose stone slide that is extremely unstable and is actually a stone avalance or slide area). If you make it you're on your way and if you don't you will slide to your death over the cliffs and jagged rocks below, or at least your boots, clothes and perhaps your body will be severely cut up by the sharp scree rocks. Only a fool would try it, and these fools die each year in similar situations. Go back, pick another safer route and live to see another day.

One good method of walking out, if applicable to your particular situation, is following a waterway. This is a good system to use especially if you have absolutely no idea of where you are. If you find a small stream carrying a substantial amount of water, it will most likely keep growing in size as you travel downstream. This small stream will probably intersect with a larger stream or river. This is what is called a confluence. Most habitations, villages, etc. are built at these confluences and this is something good to remember. You will next follow this larger river down-stream until it forms a confluence with an even larger river an so on. Sooner or later you will probably come across an inhabited cabin or village.

There are several reasons why it is especially smart to follow a waterway as mentioned. First of all, and most important, is you are following your precious water supply and dehydration will not be a problem to you. Chances are there will be fish somewhere in this water system so always stop and fish the most likely spots as shown in the fishing chapter. Animals also need this precious water for their daily needs and they will be close to it. This again improves your chances of food procurement. A good share of your edible plants will be growing along these streams and rivers (see plant chapter). If you take your time and use your head you will probably be all right using this system. Also as the water becomes larger it may very well be used as a land mark for bush pilots, so have your signals ready.

If you find yourself in the high mountains your best move will be to take the time to survey the entire area around you. Look for a valley that will probably have a small stream or river to start from. Pick a safe route down to it. Take your time and get there alive. Once you get there, start following that stream. Traveling in high mountain country can be dangerous, you may not find water readily and small game may be scarce. Usually the easiest path down out of the mountains is a game trail. Big game such as a moose will always choose a safe, easy way. This is a good trail to walk on and it will probably sooner or later, lead you directly to water.

I'd like also to clarify a very important point here. When traveling next to waterways, don't even consider building a raft and floating it. If you don't know the waterway, consider it dangerous. I've spent many a day canoeing and kayaking white water and some very calm rivers can turn into white water graveyards within the blink of an eye. These waters will take boats that are made to take the abuse and turn them into splinters. I can't even imagine what it would do to an unmaneuverable raft.

Our rivers of the north are fast, cold, and dangerous. They are loaded with sweepers that will capsize almost any vessel and hold you and the boat under water permanently, rocks that can tear you and your boat to pieces in a matter of seconds and there are holes on the other side of what we call pillows that will eat boats. Again I must stress, to consider rafting these waters you aren't familiar with is insanity. Don't attempt it and stay alive. Walking takes longer but at least you'll get to where you're going in one piece.

Don't let any arm chair amateur survivalist, or novice boater tell you any different. I've had the pleasure and opportunity to kayak rivers with expert northern kayakers and not one will attempt any river unless he or she has looked it over well from beginning to end, before even thinking of putting a boat in. These real experts never take chances they don't have to, and they know exactly what they are doing before they start out. They enjoy the water, but they respect it; so should you.

If you must walk out of high mountain country in winter, you probably will face great danger from avalanches. If you find yourself on a high ridge, stay absolutely off cornices (see figure # H-2). These will break off under your weight and take you to your death. Cornices are found on sharp wind-whipped ridges.

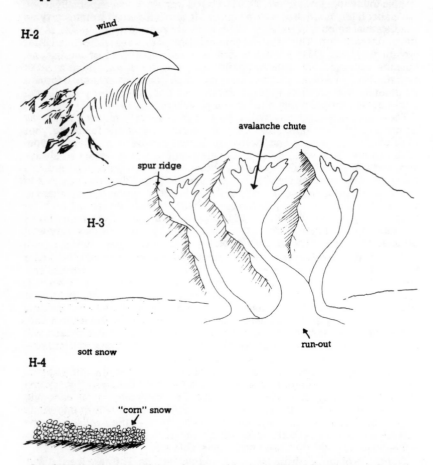

In choosing a route down from a ridge, **never** walk down a draw in winter. These are avalanche chutes. Your footsteps can trigger a massive avalanche. Always try to walk down a spur ridge. When traveling in the mountains in winter, always watch above you. Calculate where an avalanche would likely travel–they are powered by gravity and will fall along the path of least resistance. Even when you make it down to the main valley stay away from possible avalanche run-outs (see figure # H-3).

Some snow conditions are more likely than others to produce avalanches. Punch or dig through the snow to see the different layers. A lot of soft snow on top of an old crust or layer of corn snow (see figure # H-4) make avalanches very likely and very easy to trigger. However, anytime there is a lot of snow and steep slopes, consider avalanches a serious threat and avoid them.

The key here is not memorizing a lot of facts, but to be on a constant lookout and think logically about how a heavy mass would be likely to travel. A very important thing to remember here is avalanches are very fast and you can't outrun one, especially when in deep snow.

CHAPTER # 12
Direction Finding

If you have made the decision to walk out you will want to know what direction you are traveling, that is, are you traveling north, south, east, west or any variation of that? In this chapter I do not intend to give a complete lesson on orienteering and map reading. I do wish however, to cover in-depth what you will have to know in a non-planned survival situation whether or not you have a compass. I've spent many days, weeks, and months in the bush and, there have been many times when I didn't know exactly where I was. When that happens it's a very real and strange feeling. If this happens to you and you really feel "lost", regain your composure and you'll be alright. I like to tell myself that I'm never lost but at the moment I just don't know where I am. This attitude is very important and is exactly what gets you out of there. If anyone that has spent any amount of time in unfimiliar bush tells you that they have never been lost or they always knew exactly where they were, I'd have to say they are full of horse feathers. It happens to the best of us, and it's very easy to get disoriented. It's what you do about it that counts.

If you have no direction finding equipment with you at all, it's a simple matter to tell direction. One of the best methods used is the shadow stick. If there is sunlight this simple method will lay out a complete stationary compass for you and also will tell you local apparent noon. In figure # K-1 you can see how the shadow stick should be set up and how it works. This shadow stick can also help you find your latitude and longitude. In this text we are taking for granted you have no map so we will not elaborate on latitude and longitude. What is extremely important is the fact that you now have made a fine compass and you know exactly what direction north, south, east and west are. This will enable you to know what direction you are walking and help you keep walking in that direction in a straight line.

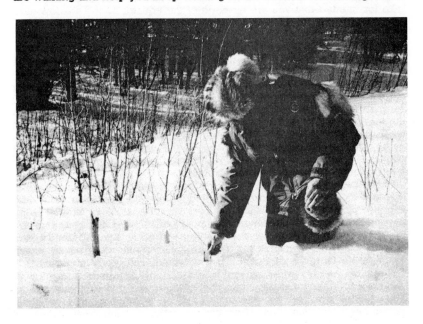

In figure # K-1 you can see and identify the shortest shadow. Set your shadow stick up in the morning and mark the ends of the shadow that's cast on the ground several times during the day. The shortest of these shadows will be local apparent noon and also your north-south line. A straight line drawn intersecting the shadow end marks will be your east-west line. The latitude you are at will dictate whether the sun is north or south of you. North of 23.4 degrees N. (latitude) the sun will always be due south at local ap-

K-1

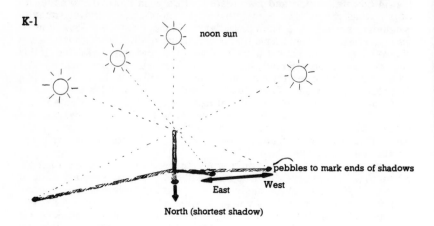

noon sun

pebbles to mark ends of shadows

East   West

North (shortest shadow)

parent noon, and thus the shadow cast at this point is showing you due north. If you are south of latitude 23.4 degrees S the sun will be north of you and the shortest shadow cast will be in the direction of due south.

Because we are concerned with northern survival in this book we will take for granted that you are far north of the equator so the shadow at its shortest point will be cast to the north. Knowing these facts, your shadow stick has just made you a very accurate compass and you now know what direction you will be traveling after you decide where you want to go.

The compass we have just made tells you what you need to know just as well as an expensive commerciall type compass. The commercial compasses have the advantage however of being portable and will work with or without the sun. One thing you must always remember about a commercial magnetic compass is the degree of declination for the area you are in. Your compass needle will point to magnetic north which, is not necessarily true north. This phenomenon is called declination or variation. This variation can be as drastic as 30 degrees east in parts of Alaska to 20 degrees west in Maine. If you have a map of the area you are in and do not allow for this declination, you can get into big trouble.

For instance, let's say you are in northern Alaska and you have a good map and compass, but you do not allow for the declination of your area which is 30 degrees east. Whatever your distance of travel may be, each degree of variation will produce an error of 1/30 of the total distance traveled. At this rate, if you travel one mile you will be ½ mile off course (see figure # K-2). As you can see when using a magnetic compass for exact direction knowing the declination in your area is extremely important.

Again we are not concerned with map and compass direction as much as we are with walking a straight line. If we are just trying to walk that straight line, declination can be discounted. Even without a shadow stick, remember that the sun travels from the east in the morning towards the west

96

in the evening. So, simply, if you put where the sun rises on your right side and where it sets on your left you will be facing north and your back will be to the south. Nature again shows us the way; this time the sun is our guide.

During periods of darkness the North Star can be our compass and path finder. The north star, properly called Polaris, is always within 1 degree from the true north pole. Again, here we are talking about the Northern

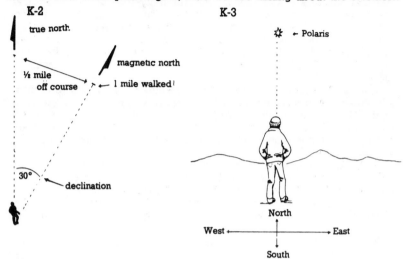

Hemishere and this is a very accurate way to get a true north reading. No matter where you are in the north, if you identify the north star, you will be looking true north within one degree. At this point you will know where east, west and south also are, and again you have created a stationary and very accurate compass (see figure # K-3).

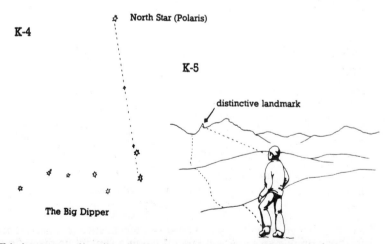

This important direction finding star can easily be found by first locating what is commonly called the Big Dipper, and then locating the two stars on its outer edge (see figure # K-4). These two stars point almost directly to the north star. The north star will be approximately five times the distance between the two reference stars of the Big Dipper. Once you have located the

North Star, forget about the Big Dipper, which like all the rest of the stars except Polaris, rotate across the sky. True north is found by facing squarely at the North Star irrespective of all other stars.

As you line up with the North Star you have just found, you will be facing due north with the south behind you, east will be at your right shoulder and west at your left shoulder. Again nature has helped you build a fine compass and this time the compass is you. Naturally, the further north you are, the closer overhead the north star will be. This is because it is a shorter sighting plane which allows a greater chance for human error if you are not careful. Take the time to line up exactly with it and you will be looking directly north. Mark this direction down on the ground with sticks or some other objects for the next day because you don't want to be traveling at night.

Now that you can indentify compass direction either by day or night and you know which direction you plan to travel, you must be able to walk a straight line in that direction. We call this procedure reference point walking. If you are walking in mountain or forest areas you will only be able to average about one mile in 40 minutes so don't over-estimate the distance you have traveled.

When you start out in a certain direction, pick out a land mark (see figure # K-5). As you walk towards that landmark, keep it in the same place in relation to you, and you will be walking in a straight line in the direction you originally chose. When you arrive at and pass your reference point you should re-check your direction with a compass, shadow stick, or the North

K-6

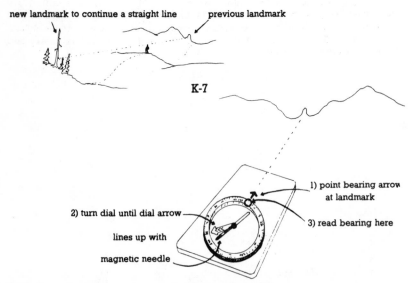

new landmark to continue a straight line   previous landmark

K-7

2) turn dial until dial arrow

lines up with

magnetic needle

1) point bearing arrow at landmark

3) read bearing here

Star and proceed on with a new reference point in view and the old one at your back. In this way you will keep walking a straight line (see figure # K-6).

If you have a magnetic compass with you, by all means use it. It is an excellent way to walk a straight line. I carry one in my survival kit and another in my jacket pocket. I use the Silva Type 3 which is an excellent compass and moderately priced. When you want to use a compass such as the Type 3 to walk a straight line without reference to maps, you can use field bearings exclusively. When you choose your reference point or field bearing (see figure # K-7). Point the bearing arrow of the compass in that precise direction. Next, turn the compass dial so as to line up the dial arrow with the red or north part of the magnetic pointer.

At this point you should also read the bearing on the dial in case it gets moved during transit and handling. From this point on all you need do at any time is line up the needle with the pre-set dial arrow and walk in the direction the bearing arrow points. This will keep you walking in a straight line toward your destination. If you have a map but don't know the declination for your area, set up a shadow stick and mark out your stationary compass. Next, compare your magnetic compass with it. You will see a difference and that difference is the declination.

Adjust the magnetic compass to be the same as your shadow stick compass and your problem is solved. Your magnetic compass now will show you a true bearing. Whenever taking a reading with your magnetic compass always try to keep it level for the readings. A magnetic compass is a precision direction finding instrument and should be treated as such. Don't abuse it and it will work for you when you need it.

Important Things to Remember

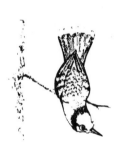

* The sun rises in the east and sets in the west.
* The shortest shadow cast from the shadow stick tells you north and south.
* When using a magnetic compass to find exact direction, declination must be known for your area.
* The North Star (Polaris) is always within 1 degree of True North.
* Always use landmarks when attempting to walk in a straight line.
* When using a magnetic compass, keep it away from metals when you are taking your reading.

CHAPTER # 13

Improvised Survival Tools & Weapons

As you know, when you're in a survival situation and your equipment is limited, you will have to improvise tools and/or weapons. Some may be simple in construction while others may become very intricate. These tools and weapons will vary because of your particular situation, requirements and materials you have at hand. In this chapter we will deal with a variety of tools and weapons that may or may not be applicable to your individual situation. My intent is to show you a way of approaching tool and weapon improvisation. The best tool for your particular need will be the one you design that will work for you.

One of the simplest and most primitive tools you might fashion would be a club. It is the best tool for clearing the branches from spruce trees for winter shelter building. A club two to two and one half inches in diameter and about two and one half feet long is perfect for me. An ax will not do a better job and you are taking the chance of cutting your leg or foot. I don't like to be repetitious, but this is an important point to remember. There are entirely too many injuries each year from an ax or hatchet. When checking your snares and deadfalls this same club can be used to finish off a poorly caught animal. This simple tool can also be used as a weapon to take slow moving small game. A club may be a simple tool but it can be very useful.

A simple spear can help you procure fish and game. A simple sharpened stick can do the job or it can be improved upon to either do a better job or a special job. At the same time, a strong, well-built spear will make a fine walking stick. In figure # N-1 you see a simple spear made from a piece of alder. It merely has one end sharpened. This will work for some applications but its major disadvantage is the point will break or dull easily. In figure # N-2 you can see an improvement made by affixing a spear head made of antler, or animal bone to it. The antler, which is bone material, can be honed to a sharp point and keen edges. The sharpening process can be accomplished by using a rough stone first and a smoother stone later. This type of improvised spear point has both penetration and cutting capability.

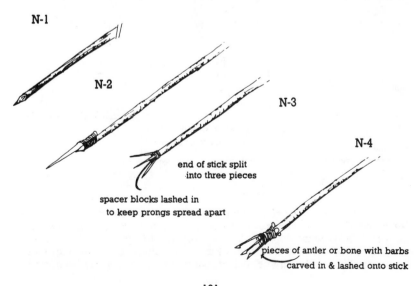

N-1

N-2

N-3

end of stick split
into three pieces

spacer blocks lashed in
to keep prongs spread apart

N-4

pieces of antler or bone with barbs
carved in & lashed onto stick

In figure # N-3 again we have a spear but this time it is designed to catch and hold a fish. It is made of wood but note that it has three prongs at different angles to both make it easier to hit the fish and then help hold the fish. This type spear can be improved upon by using bone (see figure # N-4). In the illustration you can see the prongs now have barbs on them which when used on a fish will give you more holding power. A knife can be made from bone or a piece of glass (see figure # N-5a and b). If you have some nylon cord a fine bola can be fashioned (see figure # N-6). When thrown properly at an animal's legs it will entangle them and bring the animal down.

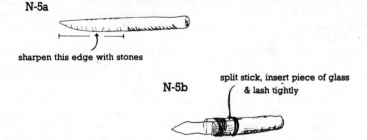

N-5a

sharpen this edge with stones

N-5b

split stick, insert piece of glass
& lash tightly

Just a simple stone can become a fine hammer to do chores around your camp or trap line. Sewing needles for repair work can be made from slivers of bone. Fish hooks can be made from wood or bone. In my survival kit, I have a sling shot rubber, and pouch. When attached to a "y" branched piece of wood I have a good sling shot (see figure # N-7). The ammunition for the sling shot can be stones or even pieces of wood. You can fashion a sling like David used to kill Goliath from a piece of cloth. A sling can hurl a fairly heavy stone a considerable distance at a tremendous rate of speed, and with practice you can be very accurate. A simple log can be a lever to move or lift a larger one. Your club can be used like a crowbar.

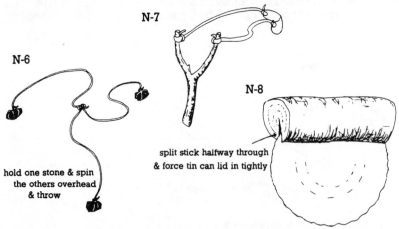

N-7

N-6

N-8

hold one stone & spin
the others overhead
& throw

split stick halfway through
& force tin can lid in tightly

As you can see, almost anything around you can be used as is, or be fashioned into a useful improvised tool or weapon. When you find the need for a tool, think what store-bought tool you would use. Then look around and improvise a similar tool from your surroundings. Be a scavenger; collect everything you can; you will probably find a use for it. And don't be restricted by conventional thinking. For instance, a fish hook and line is designed to catch fish but a baited fish hook and line can also be used to catch a bird. That used rifle cartridge you found becomes a fine whistle if you blow across it at the proper angle, or when polished and attached to a hook becomes a fishing lure. And that old tin can lid when fitted with a wooden handle becomes a sharp ulu knife (see figure # N-8).

When in deep snow, improvised snowshoes will become a necessary tool. Most people know what snowshoes are but I've talked to many people that don't really understand why they work. When walking, all your weight is being supported on a rather small surface area: the soles of your boots. This works fine on steady hard ground, but when walking in deep snow, a new problem arises. The deep snow will give way and your feet can punch through the surface right to the ground.

Without an improvised walking system such as snowshoes, walking becomes impossible and/or dangerous. Your clothes will get wet, you will be expending far too much energy, and you can find yourself in a situation where you just can't get out. In this situation you can't change your body weight but you can increase the surface area your weight rests on. When this is properly done you will be able to easily walk on top of the snow and stay dry. Snowshoes are an excellent way of accomplishing this and they can be improvised from a disabled aircraft or from natural products.

N-9   N-10

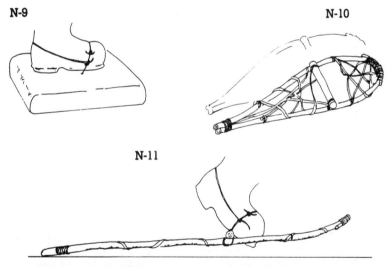

N-11

In figures # N-9 & N-10 you will see two such examples of improvised snowshoes. In figure # N-9 aircraft seats are being used as snowshoes and in figure # N-10 branches from alder or willow are fashioned into snowshoes. This particular design is similar to my regular trail shoes and will allow you to walk at a good rate of speed with little effort. When you walk with snowshoes, the binding should hinge at the toe and you will be dragging the tail end (see figure # N-11). It is not necessary to lift the whole snowshoe off the snow. These are two examples of improvised snowshoes; your situation and materials at hand may give you a completely different design but the principle will be the same.

CHAPTER # 14

Plants and Miscelaneous Edibles

Throughout the world are wild plants that may be edible, medicinal or poisonous. This chapter will cover only those that are found widely distributed across the north. All plants here are given with their Latin name so you can cross-reference them with local literature. In any given area there will be many more useful plants and for further information you should ask your local county extension service or state university horticulture department for booklets on plants.

There are many species of mushrooms in the north but unless you have already learned to identify poisonous and edible mushrooms in the specific area you are in, a survival situation is no time to experiment with edible fungi. Even edible mushrooms often do not agree with certain people and may make one person moderately ill while most people might enjoy that same mushroom with no bad effects. Mushrooms have very limited nutritional value and unless you are already very familiar with them, they are not worth the risk of dehydration, weakness and nutritional loss that will occur if you spend a day or two with vomitting and diarrhea from eating the wrong one. Some mushrooms are deadly so eat fungi only if you are very good at identifying them BEFORE you find yourself in a survival situation. For this reason, mushrooms will not be covered in this chapter.

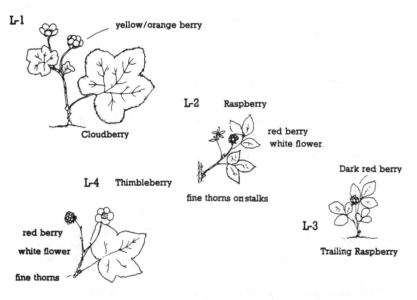

L-1 yellow/orange berry

Cloudberry

L-2 Raspberry
red berry
white flower.
fine thorns on stalks

L-4 Thimbleberry
red berry
white flower
fine thorns

Dark red berry

L-3
Trailing Raspberry

The most obvious edible wild plants are berries. Berries contain a lot of fructose, an excellent quick energy source, plus many vitamins (notably Vitamin C) and minerals. Most berries are edible, many are delicious, but some are very poisonous, so BE SURE. Cloudberry (Rubus chamaemorus), raspberry (Rubus idaeus), trailing raspberry)Rubus arcticus) and thimbleberry (Rubus parviflorus) are similar-looking and widespread. They are delicious fruits and the leaves may be cooked and eaten or a good tea made from them.

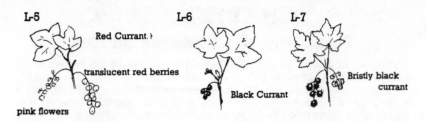

L-5 Red Currant.

translucent red berries

pink flowers

L-6

Black Currant

L-7

Bristly black currant

Currants (Ribes triste) are very good berries and the leaves are also a good tea or cooked greens Some close relatives, the black currant (Ribes hudsonianum) and the bristly black currant (Ribes lacustre) are not particularly tasty but are edible.

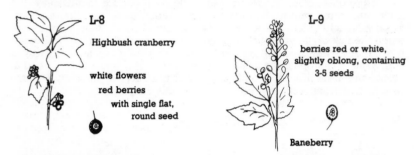

L-8

Highbush cranberry

white flowers
red berries
  with single flat,
    round seed

L-9

berries red or white, slightly oblong, containing 3-5 seeds

Baneberry

Highbush cranberry (Viburnum edule) has an acid taste but is nutritious. It can be confused with baneberry (Actaea rubra) which is very poisonous. Note that the cranberries, like currants, are in a clump which hangs down from a branch. The baneberries are located on an erect spike. A general rule to keep you out of trouble if you are not very familiar with wild plants, is don't eat berries that are on erect spikes, unless you positively can identify them as an edible species and not baneberry. Baneberries are usually red but sometimes may be white.

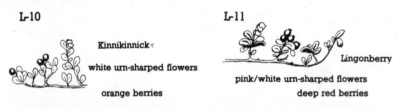

L-10

Kinnikinnick

white urn-sharped flowers

orange berries

L-11

Lingonberry

pink/white urn-sharped flowers
deep red berries

Kinnikinnik (Arctostaphylos uva-ursi) is small shrub that sprawls across the ground in dry, sandy soils all across the north. The orange-red berries are somewhat dry and flavorless but good food and one of the fruits of the north that may be found even in the winter as you dig through snow down to ground level. The leaves have traditionally been used as a tea but they have a diuretic affect (increasing urination) so the leaves should not be used in a situation where dehydration might be a problem.

Another berry commonly found all across the north, especially on sandy soils and mountainsides is the lingonberry (Vaccinium vitis-idaea), also called lowbush cranberry. Like the kinnikinnik, it is a ground-sprawling shrub and its berries are available from the end of summer throughout the winter under the snow. Lingonberries are dark red to burgundy color when ripe and considerably more juicy and tasty than the kinnikinnik. The two can be told apart by the flat paler green leaves of the kinninkinnik and the dark, shiney green leaves with slightly rolled-under edges of the lingonberry. Both are very good for you so if the two get mixed together, no harm is done.

Bog cranberries (Oxycoccus mircocarpus and Oxycoccus palustris) are commonly found in northern bogs. They have thready stems lying on the ground and tiny leaves but sizable berries that are good-tasting and nourshing.

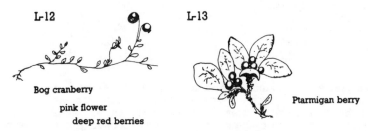

L-12

Bog cranberry

pink flower

deep red berries

L-13

Ptarmigan berry

Ptarmigan berries (Arctostaphylus alpina and Artostaphylus rubra) are also called alpine bearberries because they are a favored food of bears in the fall in the high country. The ripe berries are either red or black, very juicy, moderately good tasting and nourishing. In the fall the leathery leaves turn a brilliant scarlet color and these bright patches on a mountainside signal you from great distance that there is food there.

Crowberries (Empetrum nigrum) grow in wet areas and alpine bogs in all northern areas. They have many common names in different localities. The plant is a low, sprawling shrub and the berries are usually black, sometimes purplish, rarely white. They are juicy, tasty and very good for you.

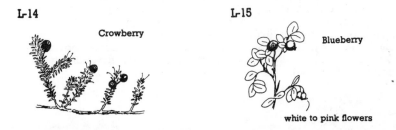

L-14

Crowberry

L-15

Blueberry

white to pink flowers

One of the most popular wild berries in most of the north is the blueberry (Vaccinium ulginosum, Vaccinium ovafolium and Vaccinium caespitosum). Different species and subspecies of the blueberry are found throughout the northern latitudes in bogs, woods and sandy mountain slopes. They are identified by their fairly small, flat leaves and berries that are dark blue, almost black, with a paler blue "blush" much like a farm-grown plum will have when ripe. The berries will have a small papery remnant of the flower still attached. They are sweet, juicy and an excellent food.

The twisted stalk (Streptopus amplexifolius), also called cucumber plant, mandarin berry or watermelon berry grows in wet areas across much of the north. The ripe berry is large, red, juicy and sweet. The green berry looks and tastes like tiny cucumbers. The stalk tastes like cucumber and is very tasty and nourishing.

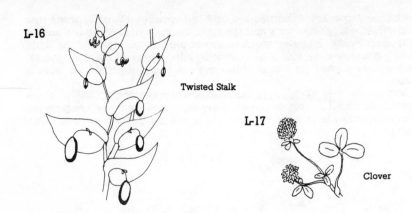

L-16

Twisted Stalk

L-17

Clover

The greatest abundance of wild edible plants in the north will be those that are eaten as raw or cooked greens. Vitamin C content as well as certain of the B vitamins will be greatest in raw plants, but Vitamin A and some minerals will be more available for absorbtion in cooked greens. If you boil plants, drink the water they were boiled in. Many valuable nutrients pass very quickly from the plant to the cooking water and it would be foolish to throw this away. The exception here is certain plants like cowslip that may be too bitter to be palatable or even mildly poisonous before boiling, but give off these bitter substances to the cooking water which then should be discarded.

Growing almost everywhere in the temperate and northern latitudes are various species of clover (Trifolium _____). Both the leaves and flowers of these plants can be eaten raw, cooked or steeped as a tea. To obtain maximum nourishment, you ought to try to eat some raw and some cooked plants of whatever kind you are finding every day.

Wild roses of various species (Rosa _____) also inhabit much of North America. The fruit has long been known as an excellent source of Vitamin C, but is also a sweet, high energy food. The leaves are sweet and tasty either raw or lightly boiled. The petals of the flowers are good in a wild salad or steeped for tea. (Steeped means held in hot but not boiling water. Many flowers and delicate green lose much of their flavor and medicinal properties if boiled).

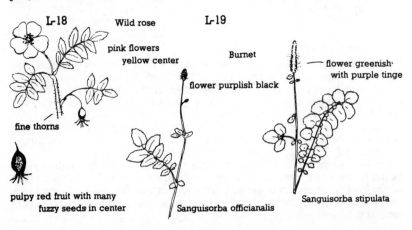

L-18   Wild rose   L-19

pink flowers
yellow center

Burnet

flower greenish·
with purple tinge

flower purplish black

fine thorns

pulpy red fruit with many
fuzzy seeds in center

Sanguisorba officianalis

Sanguisorba stipulata

Burnet (Sanguisorga officianalis and Snaguisorba stipulata) grows in moist soil and the leaves make good salad or cooking greens. Fireweed (Epilobium angustifolium, Epilobium latifolium) is also called willow herb. Species angustifolium grows in burned over areas, gravel banks or almost anywhere it can get a lot of sun. Species latifolium grows mostly on gravel/-sand bars along rivers and streams. The young leaves of both are edible but not particularly delicious. The mature leaves, especially as they begin to be tinged with red in late summer, are not very digestable. The flowers are edible and have been used rubbed on a sprained or injuried muscle to relieve soreness. The roots can be eaten raw, boiled or baked.

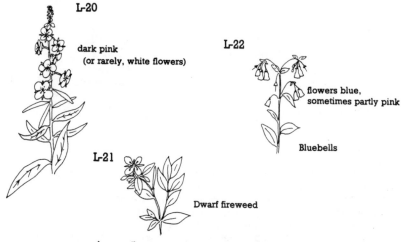

L-20

dark pink
(or rarely, white flowers)

L-22

flowers blue,
sometimes partly pink

Bluebells

L-21

Dwarf fireweed

leaves silvery-green flowers dark pink (rarely, white)

Blue bells (Mertensia paniculata) have leaves that can be eaten lightly boiled. The raw leaves are slightly fuzzy and disagreeable. The younger the leaves the better they will taste, but none are as sweet as the greens you may be accustomed to eating. Some wild foods are real taste treats but some are barely palatable. However in a survival situation, you would be very foolish to turn down any food that is safe and nourishing. There are many plants that may go by the name "blue bell" so be careful to identify it by the accompanying drawing or cross-reference it by Latin name with a book on the plants of your specific area. This is true for ALL plants. Common names vary from one locality to another. BE SURE OF A PLANT'S IDENTITY.

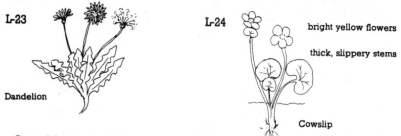

L-23

Dandelion

L-24

bright yellow flowers

thick, slippery stems

Cowslip

One of the most widespread of all plants in North America is the common dandelion. There are many species and subspecies of dandelion (Taraxacum _____) and all provide edible greens: good raw if the leaves are young, excellent boiled. Very old leaves may be very bitter and will taste better if the water they are boiled in is discarded. The flowers are good to eat raw; the roots are good baked or boiled. The dandelion is very nourishing and has been a favorite of people practicing herbal medicine for centuries. The dandelion is easy to identify and a great friend to find.

Cowslip (Caltha palustris) is found in marshes, pond edges and slow-moving streams and is characterized by thick stems, kidney-shaped leaves and yellow flowers. The leaves and stems are best eaten when young, before the flowers appear, but in any case, must be boiled before eating to destroy a poison called "helleborin". The roots are eaten boiled.

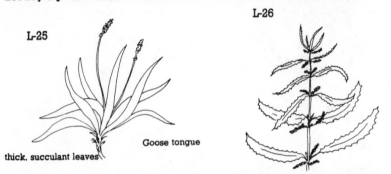

L-25

L-26

Goose tongue

thick, succulant leaves

A common plant along many seashore areas is goosetongue (Plantago maritima). The leaves and sometimes the rootstock is eaten, usually after boiling. It is an excellent choice for maintaining electrolyte balance.

Many nettles, particularly Urtica gracilis, are edible and common along northern streams and moist places. It must be boiled lightly to get rid of the irritating "fuzz". The young leaves and buds are quite good eating and very rich in many vitamins and minerals. The stinging caused by handling the raw plants can be neutralized by rubbing with either alcohol or the brown "chaff" found on the lower sections of many types of ferns.

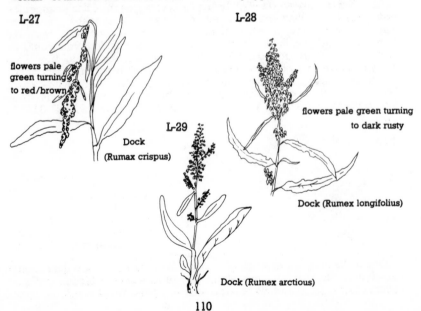

L-27

flowers pale green turning to red/brown

Dock
(Rumax crispus)

L-28

flowers pale green turning to dark rusty

Dock (Rumex longifolius)

L-29

Dock (Rumex arctious)

Many species of sorrel or dock inhabit wet places across the north. Some are native and many are introduced from Europe. Rumex crispus, Rumex longifolius, Rumex arcticus, Rumex fenestratus and Rumex mexicanus are the most widespread. Like almost all greens, they are best when the leaves are young and tender. All Rumex contain oxalic acid which may aggravate rheumatism and when the plant begins to turn deep red in late summer, will make it unpalatable or even mildly toxic. The young leaves, however, are rich in vitamins and minerals and quite good.

Mountain sorrel (Oxyria digyna) is also found in moist sheltered places. The leaves may be eaten raw for a very good source of vitamin C. They have a distinctive sour taste which increases with maturity.

A distinctive plant of the waste places, gravel bars and disturbed soils, Strawberry blite (Chenopodium capitatum) is identified by its arrowhead-shaped leaves and round deep red flowers. The leaves have a delicate spinach flavor and can be eaten raw or lightly boiled.

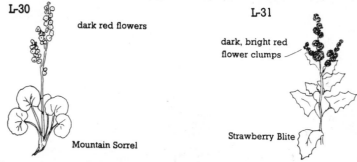

L-30

dark red flowers

Mountain Sorrel

L-31

dark, bright red
flower clumps

Strawberry Blite

There are several related plants that are commonly called pigweed or lambsquarter, the most widespread northern varieties being (Chenopodium rubrum, Chenopodium album and Chenopodium Berlandieri) introduced weeds. They are found mostly in gravelly or disturbed soils. It is characterized by its dusty green color. The leaves are excellent when picked young and lightly boiled.

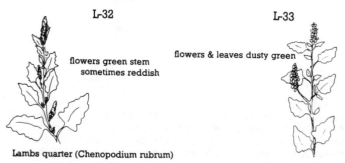

L-32

flowers green stem
sometimes reddish

Lambs quarter (Chenopodium rubrum)

L-33

flowers & leaves dusty green

Lambs quarter (Chenopodium album)

A small plant of northern peatbogs, the sundew (Drosera anglica and Drosera rotundifolia) is an insect-eater. The reddish leaves with tiny projections tipped with clear sticky syrup are sweet and improve the flavor of some of the less palatable plants you may have to eat.

The succulent leaves and stems of the roseroot (Sedum rosea), also called rosewort or stonecrop, are excellent eaten either raw or boiled, but are sweeter and more tender before the dark red flower clumps appear. The

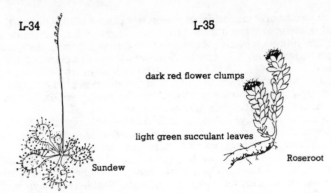

L-34

L-35

dark red flower clumps

light green succulant leaves

Sundew

Roseroot

rootstock can be eaten also and is quite good tasting when toasted or fried. It grows in rocky or gravelly soil.

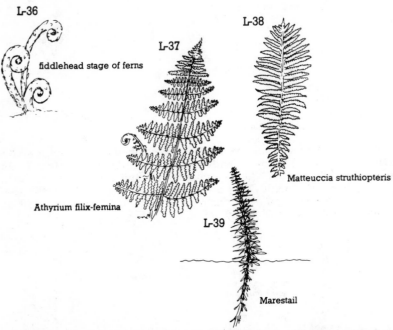

L-36

fiddlehead stage of ferns

L-37

L-38

Matteuccia struthiopteris

Athyrium filix-femina

L-39

Marestail

Many northern ferns are edible, especially in the "fiddlehead" stage when the plant first erupts from the ground and is tightly curled. Some of the widespread species that are of particular interest are the lady fern (Athyrium filis-femina), ostrich fern (Matteuccia struthiopteris), wood fern (Dryopteris dilata or spinulosa) and bracken (Pteridium aquilinum). Most ferns will be found in moist woods and meadows. The underground rootstalks are also eaten. Many natives bake and peel these rootstalks and consider them a delicacy. Some mature ferns, especially bracken are toxic.

Mares tail (Hippuris vulgaris) is found in shallow ponds and streams. It is usually eaten boiled and adds salt to the diet along with a few vitamins. It can sometimes be found sticking out of the ice on ponds or streams that are frozen but swept clear of snow and can be very valuable in maintaining an electrolyte balance if you are generating water from snow.

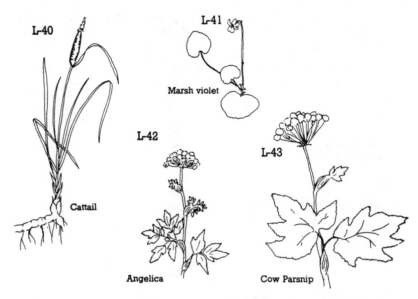

L-40 Cattail

L-41 Marsh violet

L-42 Angelica

L-43 Cow Parsnip

Cattails (Typha latifolia) are common and easy to spot in most of the north. The young stems and the flower spike while it is still green, can be eaten raw. The underground rootstalks are very starchy and an excellent energy food. The rootstalks are usually baked or boiled. Look for cattails in marshes and along the edges of ponds.

Marsh violets (Viola epipsila and Viola renifolia) are found in marshes, wet woods and along steams. Both the leaves and flowers are eaten raw and have a pleasant sweet taste. They provide a variety of vitamins and minerals.

Wild celery (Angelica lucida) and cow parsnip (Heracleum lanatum) are both found in moist areas. The young stalks are peeled and sometimes eaten raw but both taste better if cooked. The young leaves of Angelica are eaten boiled. Before eating either of these plants, BE SURE YOU CAN DISTINGUISH THEM FROM WATER HEMLOCK which is extremely poisonous. (See section on poisonous plants). Inhaling smoke of burning angelica roots is an Eskimo cure for seasickness.

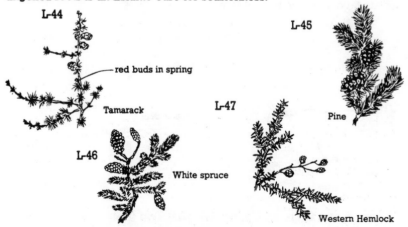

L-44 red buds in spring — Tamarack

L-45 Pine

L-46 White spruce

L-47 Western Hemlock

113

Tamarack (Larix larcina) is a small tree that lives in low, wet areas. It has needles and cones like pines, spruce and other conifers, but the tamarack needles turn yellow and drop off the trees in the fall just like deciduous trees. The young needles of the tamarack are delicious and nutritious raw or lightly boiled. The mature needles are also edible but they will become less palatable and less nutritious as they get older.

The sap and inner bark of all pines, spruce, fir and Western Hemlock is edible and an excellent source of energy food, vitamins and minerals. Some species will taste better than others but you will want to take advantage of whatever is available. The fresh sap of these trees also is an excellent wound dressing. It will close and protect the wound, make a barrier against dirt and bacteria and soothe pain.

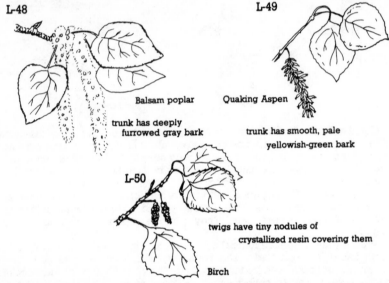

L-48

Balsam poplar

trunk has deeply
furrowed gray bark

L-49

Quaking Aspen

trunk has smooth, pale
yellowish-green bark

L-50

twigs have tiny nodules of
crystallized resin covering them

Birch

The sap and inner bark of balsam poplar (Populus balsamifera), quaking aspen (Populus tremuloides) and birch (Betula papyfera) are also edible although somewhat bitter. The sap of these trees is also a good ointment for irritated, chapped or burned skin.

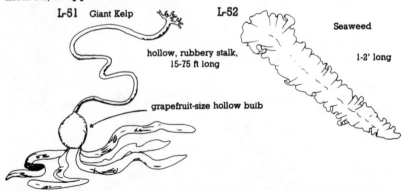

L-51   Giant Kelp

hollow, rubbery stalk,
15-75 ft long

grapefruit-size hollow bulb

L-52

Seaweed

1-2' long

Many seaweeds are edible, notably giant kelp (Nereocystis leutkeana),

114

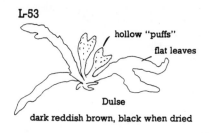

L-53

hollow "puffs"

flat leaves

Dulse

dark reddish brown, black when dried

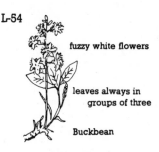

L-54

fuzzy white flowers

leaves always in groups of three

Buckbean

laver (Porphyra lacinata) and dulse (Rhodymenia palmata). Dulse is quite good tasting but all the above are excellent sources of all necesary minerals. Dried seaweed can easily be carried while you are walking and can keep your electrolyte balance steady regardless of your diet.

Buckbean (Menyanthes trifoliata) or bogbean grows in bogs and the rootstalks are starchy, providing some energy food. They are bitter and are best prepared by cutting them into small pieces and boiling several times in different water.

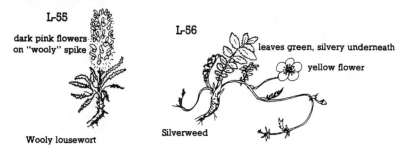

L-55

dark pink flowers on "wooly" spike

Wooly lousewort

L-56

leaves green, silvery underneath

yellow flower

Silverweed

Wooly lousewort (Pedicularis Kanei) is a common plant in dry, sandy or stoney habitats of the north. The thick root is edible raw or boiled. Another edible root is the silverweed (Potentilla anserina) which is found sprawling on sandy or rocky beaches and river bars. They can be eaten raw but are much tastier roasted or boiled.

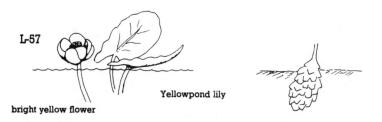

L-57

Yellowpond lily

bright yellow flower

Yellow pond lillies (Nuphar polysepalum and Nuphar variegatum), also called spatterdock, are found in ponds and slow streams that have mud bottoms. They have large thick leaves and big yellow flowers. The root bulbs that look something like pineapples and range in size from 3 to 8 inches in length are edible and a favorite food of muskrats and swans. The root is starchy and provides a high energy food. It can be eaten raw but will taste much better if it is boiled and the water discarded.

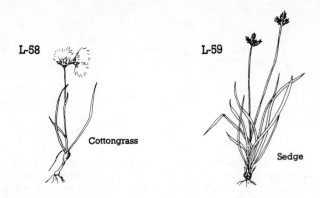

L-58 Cottongrass

L-59 Sedge

Various species of cottongrass (Eriophorum _____) grow in wet places all across the north. The root bulbs of these plants is edible and have a sweet nut-like flavor. Also growing in bogs and along the edges of stream, ponds and lakes are many varieties of sedges (Carex _____). These are course grass-like plants that also have edible root bulbs. Muskrats, voles and many other small rodents collect these bulbs and finding the food cache of one of these animals is the easiest way to obtain a substantial amount of good-tasting carbohydrate.

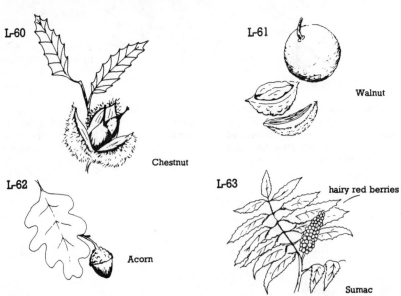

L-60 Chestnut

L-61 Walnut

L-62 Acorn

L-63 hairy red berries — Sumac

Various nuts may be found in some parts of the north. Some edible varieties are chestnut (Castanea _____), walnut (Juglans _____), beechnuts (Fagus _____) and acorns (Quercus _____). Also found in these hardwood forest environments is sumac (Rhus _____) with its edible red berries.

There are many wild plants that have been traditionally used for medicine. Some of these will serve you well in an emergency. In the water chapter we talked about the danger of dehydration which can be greatly

116

exaggerated by diarrhea, which is a frequent result of eating unfamiliar foods or foods that may be slightly spoiled. A natural cure for diarrhea that is widely available in the north is Labrador tea (Ledum palustre), also called Hudson Bay tea. A low shrub of the forests, mountains and tundra it can be positively identified by its narrow leaves that are dark green on top and fuzzy and cinnamon-colored below. A tea from the leaves (made by steeping the leaves in hot water, but not boiling) has a pungent flavor that some people like. Whether you find it agreeable or not, several cups of this will go a long ways towards curing even a severe case of diarrhea. It is reportedly toxic in large doses but many northern Indians drink it regularly with no ill affects.

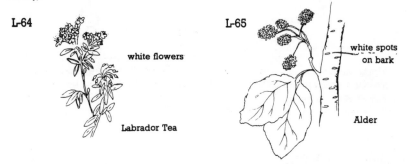

L-64

white flowers

Labrador Tea

L-65

white spots
on bark

Alder

A strong tea made by boiling the bark and inner bark of alder (Alnus crispa and Alnus incana) is very useful to wash wounds and to wash out an infected or injured eye. The alder is indentified by large toothed leaves that are dark on top and a paler green below, smooth purplish-grey bark with whitish marks (see illustration) and small cones resembling miniature pine cones.

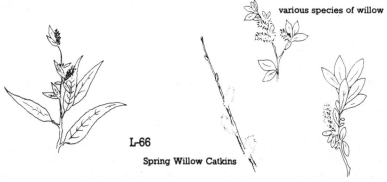

various species of willow

L-66

Spring Willow Catkins

Any shrub of the large genus of willows (Salix _____) have a substance in the inner bark called salycillin, from which aspirin was originally derived. Chewing the bark will provide a mild pain-reliever. The leaves of willows are also edible and extremely rich in vitamin C. The younger the leaves, the more tender and palatable they will be.

Yarrow (Achillea millefolium and Achillea borealis) grow almost everywhere in the north that there is sandy or gravelly soil. A tea made from the flowers (by steeping, NOT boiling) is very effective in breaking a fever. It will also help with a sore throat and to clear congestion of the respiratory tract. The flowers, when smashed and scrubbed onto the skin provide a measure of temporary insect repellance.

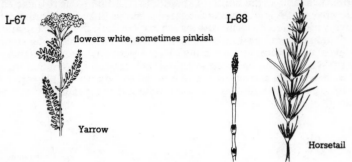

L-67

flowers white, sometimes pinkish

Yarrow

L-68

Horsetail

Horsetail (various members of the genus Equisetum) steeped in hot water provide a wash for festered wounds. Different species will be found from bogs to scree slopes. It is identified by its jointed stem and feathery, brittle leaves that have a course, almost sandpaper feel.

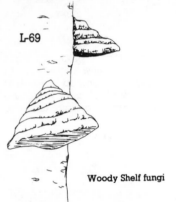

L-69

Woody Shelf fungi

Another useful group of plants are the various woody shelf fungi that grow on the trunks of old or dead trees. A few of these smoldering around your camp will give a thick and not-too-pleasant smoke that will repel flying insects. The musty smoke takes some getting used to, but when the bugs are really bad, it is well worth it.

To safely use edible plants, it is necessary to have an equal familiarity with the poisonous plants of the area. Here again, I will only cover those which are common to much of the north. Many poisonous plants are not deadly, but in a survival situation, you cannot afford the drain on your system caused by severe digestive upset, so be careful. It is always my policy that if I am not completely sure a plant is edible, to test it in several stages. First, I break the stem and touch the broken end to my tongue. If there is no burning or radically unpleasant taste, I chew and spit out a piece about the size of a dried split pea. Then I wait about 5 minutes. If there is still no negative effect, I chew and swallow a slightly larger piece. If after ten minutes or so, all seems right, I will eat a tiny bit more and wait at least 4 hours for the effect before concluding that the plant in question is edible.

The first poisonous plant I will talk about is one of the most deadly in much of the north. It is also very important because it so closely resembles several edible plants. It is water hemlock (Circuta Douglasii and Cicuta mackenzieana), a fairly common plant in wet areas. The whole plant is poisonous, but the roots contain the most concentrated poison. Water hemlock can be positively identified by slicing the root bulb vertically. If the bulb is composed of several distinct chambers, do not eat it, wash your knife and your hands thoroughly.

118

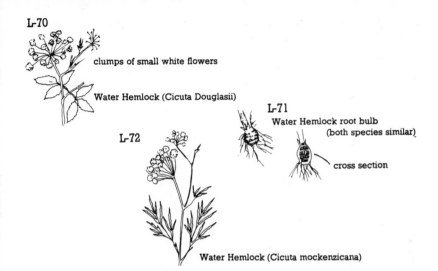

L-70

clumps of small white flowers

Water Hemlock (Cicuta Douglasii)

L-71
Water Hemlock root bulb
(both species similar)

cross section

L-72

Water Hemlock (Cicuta mockenzicana)

False hellebore (Veratrum viride and Veratrum album) grows in moist meadows. It is a tall showy plant that is very useful as shelter building material, but quite poisonous to eat.

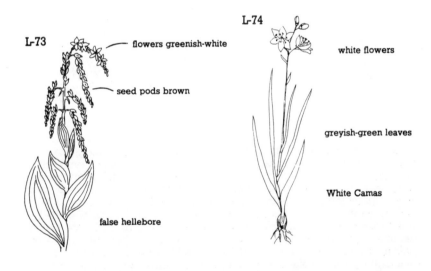

L-74

white flowers

L-73

flowers greenish-white

seed pods brown

greyish-green leaves

White Camas

false hellebore

White camas (Zygadenus elegans) is a member of the lily family that grows in open meadows and grassy slopes. The poison is found throughout the plant but is most concentrated in the root.

Larkspur (Delphinium glaucum) and monkshood (Aconitum delphinifolium) both grow in moist but drained habitats. Both contain poison which is most concentrated in the roots. Monkshood has the unique characteristic though, of being a pain reliever when the flowers or roots are rubbed on a sore joint or muscle, IF THE SKIN IS NOT BROKEN. It is highly poisonous if taken internally or applied to broken skin.

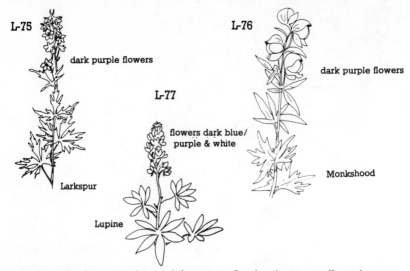

L-75 dark purple flowers

Larkspur

L-76 dark purple flowers

Monkshood

L-77 flowers dark blue/ purple & white

Lupine

Lupines (various members of the genus Lupinus) are usually poisonous, some species more than others and the poison mainly concentrated in the seeds and roots. Nightshade (Solanum nigrum) is another poisonous plant that grows primarily in well-drained soils.

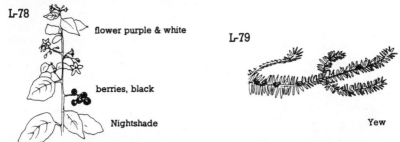

L-78 flower purple & white

berries, black

Nightshade

L-79

Yew

There are severals species of yew (Taxus _____) throughout the north and all should be considered poisonous. They are evergreen shrubs and care must be taken to not confuse them with other short-needled evergreens. First, notice that the yew needles are arranged in two flat rows along the twigs, not growing out from all around the twig. Yew have no cones, but instead bear their seeds in red berries or flat scarlet disks.

If you are dealing with plants that you are unsure of, there are several general rules to keep you on the safe side. First, there are numerous poisonous plants and very few edible ones that have dark purple flowers. The same goes for plants with deeply palmated leaves (shaped like the monkshood or larkspur leaves). There are some edible plants with this type of leaf, but if you don't know, play it safe. Thirdly, if a plant is green when young and turns all or partly red or purple with age, it is probably somewhat poisonous, at least in the stage when it has begun to change color.

Besides plants and obvious fish and game, there are many food sources in the wilderness. Most are small, hidden or strange sounding to conventional western tastes. Many of these are delicacies in other cultures or diet staples of aboriginal people. So if you're in a survival situation, you may have to put aside some food prejudices and try the following.

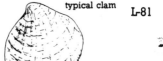

typical clam

L-81

dimple in the sand at low tide
indicates presence of a clam

L-82

clam's neck

foot-for digging

The sea coast provides an abundance of creatures to eat. An old Tlinget Indian saying goes, "When the tide goes out, the table is set". Clams may be spotted in sandy areas by watching for the dimples in the sand where their necks reach the surface. If there is a sudden movement in the dimple when you step near it, dig quickly and pull out the clam.

L-83

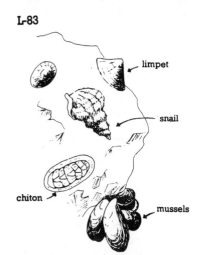

limpet

snail

chiton

mussels

Rocks along the tidal margin will be almost always covered with various molluscs. Limpets, chitons, snails and mussels can all be plucked off the rocks. They will all seperate from their shells when cooked and are very good nutrition. There has been a lot of effort in recent years by different agencies to convince people that these tidal animals are deadly to eat. A particular algae, commonly called "red tide" does occasionally move into an area and all shallow water algae-eaters such as clams and mussels will contain the toxin from this algae. Anyone eating infected shellfish will suffer from a condi-

tion known as "paralytic shellfish poisoning".

The symptoms of paralytic shellfish poisoning begin with numbness of the mouth and may end with respiratory arrest and death. Onset of symptoms is usually within minutes of eating the infected shellfish. This condition is very serious but fear of it shouldn't stop you from enjoying the abundant food of the sea coast if you are careful. The first thing to look for when considering eating tidal zone shellfish, is the other birds and animals that feed on these same molluscs. Black oystercatchers and any other large shorebirds such as whimbrels and curlews feed on molluscs and if you find any of these birds dead on the shore, you should be

L-84

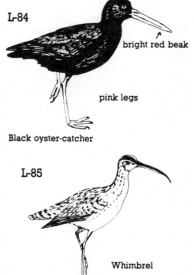

bright red beak

pink legs

Black oyster-catcher

L-85

Whimbrel

suspicious. The same would hold true for sea otters. However, there are many other possible causes of death for these animals so finding just one dead animal does not necessarily indicate presence of a red tide.

L-86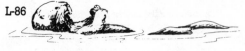

Sea Otter

If I find just one dead specimen or I see no living mollusc-eater, I would cautiously test a sample. Eating one whole purple mussel could possibly kill a person if there is a heavy infestation, so just like with testing plants, I would just touch the meat of the mussel or clam to my tongue and wait ten or fifteen minutes before chewing and spitting out a very tiny bite and waiting another 20 minutes or so. If there is no numbing sensation or other unpleasant effect, I would proceed to make a meal of some very delicious seafood. Red tide does exist, but with common sense, there is no reason to starve where for centuries the Indians have enjoyed a banquet.

Octopus can sometimes be found under large rocks at low tide. Look for piles of broken shells outside a hole under a rock. Poke into the hole with a long stick and when the octupus grabs ahold, jerk the stick out quickly. You must then stab the octopus very quickly in the head or it will escape. A more effective technique is to bait a large hook on the end of your stick and shove this in the hole, wait for the octopus to grab it, then jerk it out. The meat of an octopus is very fine eating, raw or lightly boiled. It looks rather dangerous but is actually a very shy animal.

In fresh water there are usually different kinds of snails, aquatic insects and other small invertebrates that can be gathered and cooked. In even the most barren of areas, there are usually ants, locusts, grasshoppers, lizards or frogs to eat. Under the bark of trees that show holes bored by wood-eating beetles, you can find fat white grubs that may look gross to you, but are actually not bad tasting especially if toasted. Bears and woodpeckers certainly seem to think these little creatures are delicious.

In a survival situation, you may look around and see no food at all. But remember, native people lived all over this continent long before there were farms and stores. They lived on just what is there before you and they procured it, stored it, prepared it with just those tools and materials that are available to you in the wilderness. Don't be narrow-minded about what is edible. You can be squemish and starving or sensible and well-fed and healthy.

Chapter # 15
Clothing

The clothing you happen to be wearing when you find yourself in a survival situation can have a great deal to do with how successfully you come out of the ordeal. Since a survival situation is always something you didn't plan on, it is wise to wear or carry with you good survival clothing anytime you are away from home. Even for a short trip in a car I always have with me the clothing and gear I would want if the worst possible thing should happen.

The market is flooded with all sorts of outdoor garments, some excellent, some junk and a lot in between. Some garments are very good in one type of condition but useless in most others. For survival gear, you want the most versatile items you can get because you don't know what you might encounter. You might have the warmest parka made for cold dry weather and then find yourself out in a cold rain—with hypothermia. You can't carry a truckload of clothing with you so choose carefully items that will serve in the widest variety of circumstances.

One of the biggest problems you must deal with as far as proper clothing goes, is moisture. Moisture will come from the outside as rain, snow, splashing or immersion in water, etc.; as well as from the inside from the insensible perspiration that is taking place 24 hours a day, regardless of your activity, and the sweating caused by exertion. All garments will be less warm when wet than when dry. However some fabrics are less affected by moisture than others.

In very cold conditions, moisture from the outside is negligable. The moisture you will have to contend with will be body perspiration. There are two basic theories on how to best control this moisture. The vapor barrier theory is based on wearing some sort of water-proof garment close to the skin to hold this moisture in, thereby keeping the main insulating layers of outer clothing dry and at full thermal efficiency. A good example of this is a treated nylon shirt worn under a down parka.

The other theory is to wear garments that quickly transfer moisture away from the skin and out to the air. Polypropylene underwear under a thinsulite® parka is a good example of this system since both those materials are specifically designed to pull moisture away and evaporate it. Those fabrics are also designed to perform well as insulation even when wet.

Personally, with the materials such as polypropylene and thinsulite® available today, I find the theory of keeping dry by pulling moisture away from the body to be vasty superior in the long run than the vapor barrier system. I have found that allowing the body to become wet is not only uncomfortable but can lead to very dangerous chilling. Using the "keep dry" system you must be careful to avoid excessive sweating by taking off heavy outer garments when working as soon as you feel yourself beginning to heat up.

Different fabrics have different characteristics and each should be understood so you can plan a clothing system of layers. Layering is the only practical way to approach outdoor clothing. If you are wearing a light shirt and a super-warm parka and you start working strenuously you will soon be too warm for the parka. You can take the parka off and become chilled by wearing only a light shirt (and once chilled it will be very difficult to warm back up) or you can drench your parka with sweat, making it uncomfortable and less efficient when you will really need all the warmth you can get later. Either way is not a good choice. If instead, you were wearing a light shirt, followed by a heavier shirt and/or sweater, followed by a parka, you could peel off the parka while you work in comfort and have a dry parka to get back into before you chill off.

Most commonly worn next to the skin for most people is a T-shirt. 100% cotton has the characteristic of abosorbing and holding moisture. For this reason, it would be the best choice for a first layer in the vapor barrier system but a very poor idea for a keep-dry system. Many T-shirts today are 50% cotton, 50% polyester and do not retain much moisture and do serve somewhat to transfer it to outer layers. A 50/50 T-shirt adds a very small amount of insulation to either system and has a small value.

Insulating underwear has changed profoundly over the years. In past generations wool "longhandles" were standard. Wool tends to hold moisture but dries from the inside out and for keeping its insulative value when wet, few, if any fabrics can beat it. Its disadvantage that led to its fall from popularity is that it is too scratchy to be worn next to the skin. Wool underwear lined with silk is comfortable, warm and expensive. Silk alone has substantial insulative value for a fabric that is non-bulky and close-fitting.

The wool longhandles were pretty much replaced by thermal-knit cotton which is comfortable, cheap and warm as long as it is dry. It is definitely out-classed by the newer (or older) fabrics available. Polypropylene is one of the modern fabrics that has been on the market long enough to be thoroughly tested and found excellent. It pulls moderate amounts of moisture away from the skin, maintains considerable insulative value even if soaked, dries very quickly and is very comfortable next to the skin.

The next layer of clothing will be a shirt or sweater or combination. This layer should be warm enough to work in when temperatures are moderately cold. There are many fabrics on the market, but few can equal 100% wool. Wearing cotton underneath polypropylene or as the shirt layer over it defeats the purpose of the keep-dry system. Acrylons and other synthetics may or may not add much value here, depending on how they are woven or knitted. A loose, bulky knit or weave will be warmer than a tight, thin weave. Some pre-shrunk wools such as "Dachstein" sweaters have a tight knit because they are pre-shrunk to make them more windproof, but are still very warm due to the bulk and the fact that they are 100% wool.

For summer time in northern wilderness, your outer layer will be some durable wind-proof jacket with a rain-coat or a combination storm jacket. A raincoat alone functions poorly as a windbreaker if you are walking or working strenuously because it will trap a good deal of body moisture underneath and soak your garments no matter what material they are made of. There are fabrics on the market that are supposed to be rainproof but breathable so that body moisture passes through. They work to a certain extent but my choice would be a jacket of "mountain cloth" (65% cotton, 35% nylon) and a good raincoat on the side.

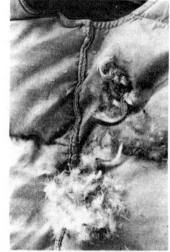

In winter, a good parka is a must. Goose down insulation has been the standard for many years and without a doubt, is the warmest, ounce for ounce, insulation commonly available. However, it has several very serious drawbacks. First, down has absolutely zero insulative value when it gets wet. It mats down considerably (and thereby loses warmth) when even dampened from moderate perspiration and it dries very slowly. It has little value if compressed and if it must be stored tightly stuffed it has a shorter useful lifespan than the good synthetic insulations available today. Down also will not draw moisture outward as part of a keep-dry system. If you use a down parka you are almost forced to use a vapor barrier system to get the most from the down insulation.

New synthetic parka insulations are constantly being introduced. Polarguard® and Holofil® are two very good ones that both will maintain insulative capacity when damp, dry quickly and pull moisture away from the body to a certain extent. After testing many insulation fabrics, my personal choice is Thinsulite® . It is the best I've found for drawing moisture away from the body. It keeps a high degree of insulation when fairly wet, dries rapidly and unlike all the others, maintains good insulative value even when compressed. Doubled 150 weight "Thinsulite" makes a parka good to 40° below zero.

The material for the parka shell is also important. It must not be a waterproof material or it will trap body moisture. External moisture is of little concern in very cold weather where you would have an occasion to wear a heavy parka. 100% nylon fabric has the disadvantage of melting quickly if a spark from a fire should land on it. 100% cotton soaks up too much moisture and if heavy enough to be very durable, weighs too much to be practical. Mountain cloth combines the best features of both, 35% nylon to give strength without bulk and the ability to pass moisture out to the air and cotton for its durability. The resulting cloth will get a hole in it if a spark hits it, but not nearly as much of one as pure nylon.

An important feature of a parka is the hood. Although under most circumstances a hood is awkward and restricts hearing and vision to an aggravating degree, when a strong, cold wind is blowing, a hood is very valuable. I prefer a hood with a ruff that is wolf on the outer strip and wolverine on the inside and can be turned up to form a fur "tunnel" to protect my face under extreme windy arctic conditions. This may not be necessary or practical for most people but it is what it takes for the worst the arctic can offer.

Another important feature of a parka is lots of pockets. It should have insulted hand-warmer pockets and large cargo pockets. I prefer to have numerous pockets inside to carry survival and medical gear and a water container.

Pants are an item taken for granted most of the time, but there are good ones and bad ones for a survival situtation. Even though denim jeans are what I normally wear, when travelling, I keep a pair of wool pants with me. Denim is a sturdy material but being made of cotton, it will soak up a tremendous amount of moisture, starting at the cuffs and "wicking" it on up your legs. It is cold when wet or in the wind. A heavy wool or wool/nylon blend is a very warm pair of pants. The tighter the weave the more windproof.

A hat is an essential part of your survival clothing. A wool watch cap is small and easy to take along but can literally save your life. A person can lose up to 40% of his body heat through an unprotected head. If you are chilled all over, simply putting on a hat can make a very noticable difference. Here again, wool is the old stand-by. Polypropylene liners for wool hats are a new development that vastly expands the value of an old favorite. Fiberpile is also an excellent choice for a hat because it will move moisture away from the skin and stay warm even in the rain. The balaclava style hat pulls down for a partial mask to protect the chin and sides of the face and also has a slight bill to keep a driving snow or rain out of your eyes.

To function in the cold, you must protect your hands. Different people have different tolerances for cold hands but you should include both gloves and warm mittens in your survival gear since you never know what conditions you might have to deal with. Again I come back to my favorite fabrics. Wool with polypropylene liners and a nylon pack cloth outer shell makes a mitten "system" that allows you to add or take off layers according to temperature. Layering also makes it easier to dry your mittens since they can be separated and spread along a rack. A pair of gloves that are heavy enough to be moderately warm but light enough to allow you free use of your fingers are essential since in very cold temperatures you do not want to be exposing your bare hands even when doing tasks that you cannot perform with mittens on. Wool and polypropylene gloves will give you the most warmth for the least bulk.

The part of the body most commonly frostbitten is the feet. The reason is not anything peculiar about our feet, but that we most often neglect them, especialy if we are not planning on being in a wilderness situation. Going someplace in a car or airplane is typical—we expect that the vehicle will safely deliver us from one sheltered environment, through the cold, to another sheltered environment with our feet all the while kept toasty warm by the vehicle's heater. But what if the vehicle fails? Now you are stranded along a highway or in the wildernes perhaps under some very austere conditions and what do you have on your feet? You likely will be wearing a reasonable coat but your street shoes provide almost no protection at all.

There are three factors to consider for warm footgear. First is insulation, second is allowing free circulation and third is keeping dry. Boots like snowmobile boots and others which have a rubberized foot, leather or nylon upper and a felt liner are very good for temperatures down to 15° or 20° below zero. They will keep external moisture out, provide moderate insulation and if they fit loosely enough, will not hinder circulation. (If your footgear, or any item of clothing, fits tightly enough to restrict circulation at all, it will be ineffective at keeping you warm no matter how much insulation it has). A warm boot with one too many pair of socks will not be very warm.

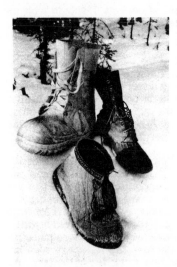

For temperatures below minus 20° the best choices of footgear are mukluks or military vapor barrier boots. Mukluks work on the principle of being soft and loose-fitting. With a good wool liner and a couple pair of wool socks, a properly designed and fitted pair of Indian or Eskimo style mukluks will be very warm.

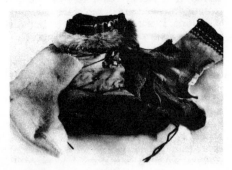

Their main liability is that they cannot be worn under wet conditions or in snow if the temperature is above zero or they will become wet. They are however, light-weight and very comfortable.

The vapor barrier boots, also called bunny boots or V B boots, are the only footgear that will for sure keep your feet warm under even the worst conditions. They are big, heavy, awkward and ugly. But they are the ultimate when things are really grim. They work on the principle of trapped air between two layers of heavy rubberized fabric. They will keep your feet warm even if you completely immerse your feet in water and then walk in minus 50° or colder. They will cause your feet to sweat and become wet inside of the boot, but in this one particular case, they are so well designed that your feet will stay warm anyway. Any other footgear very rapidly loses value as moisture from perspiration builds up.

For all other cold weather boots, you must at every opportunity, remove the liners and your socks and dry them. If you are active, you will be giving off moisture inside of your boots even when you are not aware of actual sweating. Your feet will become damp and this quickly leads to cold feet and then frostbite. Unless you are wearing bunny boots, be very careful to keep your footgear dry!

Extreme cold weather clothing is usually bulky and rarely very fashionable. When traveling in a car or plane it is uncomfortably warm to wear. But a survival situation is always the unexpected possibility and without proper clothing, you have begun with two big strikes against you. Go ahead and wear a light coat and street shoes, but by all means, carry with you what you need for the very worst that could possibly happen.

In the event that you get caught in a cold weather survival situation without the proper clothing, you will have to improvise. I can give you a few suggestions, but when it happens you will have to assess what you have available and invent ways of using what you can find. If there is a vehicle as part of your situation, it probably has foam rubber seats. Use the foam for insulation and the upholstery for the outer fabric of a pair of mukluks. Form them loosely around your feet and tie with whatever is available. Remember to tie them so that they will stay on but be loose and the foam not too compressed—once you squeeze the air spaces out of something, it is not warm. Mittens can be made in the same fashion.

Dry sphagnum moss or crushed dry leaves will serve as insulation for mittens or mukluks if you can find a piece of fabric or plastic to contain them. Certainly save and use the hide, fur and feathers of any animal you can kill and adapt it for clothing. Skins of fairly large fish can be the outer covering of makeshift boots or mittens. The dry mosses and animal hides can line a "mouse nest" style sleeping area. If you line a snow cave with spruce boughs and cover yourself with dried mosses, grass or leaves, you can sleep quite warmly. Being cold is more than a discomfort. It saps your energy and hinders your judgement. So always prepare for the worst and if it happens, improvise with everything that is available.

CHAPTER # 16

First Aid and Wilderness Medicine

This section of the book deals with both first aid and wilderness medical care. I will use the term first aid to mean that attention given to a sick or injured person temporarily because the patient will soon be in the care of a doctor and/or hospital. Unfortunately, in a wilderness survival situation there will be no doctor coming so you will have to become the doctor. This treatment we will term wilderness medicine.

There is no mystery to proper medical care and if need be you can and will have to function as your own doctor. You will need an understanding of human anatomy, how and why certain things happen in your body, what to check and how to remedy the problem. Gretchen and I are not only certified First Aid and CPR instructors, but nationally certified EMT's (Emergency Medical Technicians), and in most cases our medical work has been in the bush where there is no doctor or hospital. It is our belief that every man, woman and child in this country should be trained in first aid and CPR. So many people die each year that didn't have to because they or the people around them didn't have even a basic knowledge of first aid. It is my intention to offer you this knowledge and I hope you will relay it to your entire family. It may well save a life.

One very important thing everyone should have is a good first aid kit. You should have one in your house, one in your vehicle and one on your person whenever you are fishing, hunting, camping or traveling in the wilderness. Injuries, especially in a survival situation, must be taken care of immediately and properly. When you make up your kit, don't skimp on bandaging and dressing materials or on antibiotics. Any untended open wound is prone to infection and that is the last thing you need in a wilderness survival situation. As you make up your kit, you will probably need some help from your doctor to aquire prescription items. Once your kit is complete, keep it that way. If you use something, replace it as soon as possible. And then, don't go anywhere without it.

Section # 1—Wounds

Wounds can be classed in two major categories—open and closed. An open wound is one where the skin is actually broken and a closed wound is one where the skin is not broken but the tissue beneath it has suffered a trauma. Open wounds can be sub-classed into at least five categories: abrasions, lacerations, incisions, punctures and avulsions. Abrasions are wounds where bleeding is negligable but the outer layers of skin have been destroyed or damaged, such as a scrape or brush burn. Although this injury is minor there is danger of infection and the wound should be irrigated (washed by pouring or squirting, not by scrubbing) with sterile saline solution or clean water as soon as possible, treated with an antibacterial ointment and covered with a dressing and bandage.

The wound classed as an incision can be caused by any number of objects. In the wilderness, it is usually a knife. This type of wound is usually more serious than an abrasion because heavy bleeding may occur. Arteries and veins may be damaged along with tendons, nerves and muscles. The wound should be irrigated and the bleeding stopped. The wound should then be covered with a sterile dressing and bandage. This will suffice for first aid treatment if you will be seeing a doctor right away.

If this is a wilderness medical situation the treatment should be as follows. The wound should be irrigated with hydrogen peroxide from your kit and scrubbed with a povidone iodine pad. This will probably re-start the bleeding but is necessary. Again stop the bleeding but do not contaminate the wound. You must at this time determine how deep the wound is and how you intend to close it. If the wound is not too deep it can be closed with either butterfly bandages or steri-strips from your kit (see figure # M-1). The wound should then be coated lightly with an antibiotic ointment such as Bacitracin. Next apply a sterile gauze dressing and bandage it in place. Keep the dressing dry and change it if it becomes wet. The butterflies or steri-strips should be left in place until the wound has healed, usually about 10 days.

M-1

butterfly
closures

steri-strips

The wound we call a laceration has jagged or irregular edges. There will usually be more trauma to the tissue under the skin due to the method of injury such as falling and being cut on a jagged rock. The treatment will be the same as for an incision.

A puncture wound can be very serious. External bleeding should be encouraged to act as an irrigation cleansing process. Next, clean the wound with hydrogen peroxide followed by scrubbing with a povidone pad. Apply antibiotic ointment and a sterile dressing. If you have an oral antibiotic in your kit, now would be a good time to use it. Note however, that this or any time you use an oral antibiotic for any reason, you must take the full course. If it says take for 10 days, take it for the full 10 days; don't quit after 3 or 4 because you feel better or the wound looks OK. If you take only a partial course of antibiotic, a few hardy microbes will probably survive and you will have inadvertently develped a strain of bacteria that is resistant to the antibiotic and when you have a recurrance of the infection it will be much more severe and harder to treat.

A puncture wound, like all wounds should be checked frequently for infection. If swelling or redness around the puncture occurs, soak the wound in warm water (as hot as you can toerate) 5 times a day, at least 15 minutes each time. Clean pieces of cloth can be soaked in hot water and applied to the wound if you cannot immerse the part of the body on which the wound is located. Between soaks, apply antibiotic ointment and a sterile dressing. Hopefully this will bring the infection to the surface where it will drain safely. If the swelling continues, the puncture wound will have to be lanced to allow the pus to drain so that the toxins do not get into the bloodstream. Lancing should be done with the sterile scalpel blade from your kit. Once you have located the pus pocket, allow it to drain on its own. Never squeeze it or the infection may be driven deeper into your body. Once the abscess has been drained, continue the hot water soaks, with antibacterial ointment and a clean dressing after each soak.

An avulsion is a very serious wound. When a part of the body has been torn or cut off, or most of the way off, it is called an avulsion. Bleeding will be heavy and shock is likely to occur. For first aid, stop the bleeding, treat for shock and get immediate medical attention. Also, the avulsed part should be kept clean and cool and transported with the victim. A surgeon can often re-attach it to the body.

In a wilderness medical situation, you will not be getting to a surgeon in time to be concerned with reattachment of the avulsed part. Your primary concerns will be stop the bleeding and treat for hypovolemic shock. Once the bleeding has been stopped (see the sections on bleeding and shock), the area of the avulsion must be irrigated and disinfected, first with hydrogen peroxide and then cleaned with a povidone pad. Next apply an antibiotic ointment and cover the wound with a non-adhering dressing. Place a sterile gauze pad over the dressing and bandage securely. This disinfecting and dressing procedure must be performed each day. If you have an oral antibiotic, use it.

Each day you will have to scrub away all the yellowish or whitish crust or bits of dead tissue that appear, even though this procedure is extremely painful. The alternative is bloodpoisoning or gangrene. Either one will kill you. During this scrubbing process it is a healthy sign if the wound bleeds a little. Under no circumstance, allow the wound to scab over.

If you have a semi-avulsed wound like a finger tip or any large flap of tissue that is not completely severed from the body, you will want to irrigate, disinfect and put the tissue back in place. Then cover the wound with a sterile dressing and stop the bleeding by direct pressure (see bleeding section). Here again, the dressing must be changed daily. With each change, the wound must be disinfected and any yellowish matter removed. Within a matter of days the avulsed tissue will turn black. This hard black "carapace" is a good sign-do not remove it. It will eventually sluff off. If the semi-avulsed tissue becomes slimey, starts to smell and there is a dark red inflamation of the neighboring tissue, the semi-avulsed tissue must be removed entirely and the whole area scrubbed (with a povidone pad, preferably) until it bleeds freely. If the bleeding becomes severe, disinfect, dress and stop the bleeding by direct pressure.

You can see by this point that it is very wise to have assembled a good first aid kit and have it with you. There are alternative methods and materials offered to you in the wilderness, however. Just as with your wilderness survival skills, your wilderness medical knowledge must increase as your equipment and materials decrease. For example, if you don't have any sterile gauze dressings to cover a wound, spruce or pine pitch will effectively seal it off from outside contamination which leads to infection.

When it comes to irrigating a wound, nature can help you again. If you don't have hydrogen peroxide, clean water will do. If the water is boiled and then allowed to cool it will be sterile. Two excellent additives to sterile water are alder bark or equisetum boiled to a strong decoction, as explained in the plant chapter. These have been used for many centuries by natives and even our European ancestors.

You know the danger of infection in an open wound especially a puncture wound. The wilderness offers some excellent poultice materials. One use of a poultice is to draw the poisons (pus, etc.) from an infection that has become subcutaneous (in the deeper tissue). When the poultice draws the poison to the skin surface, you will see a white pocket just under the skin. Sometimes this pocket will burst and drain on its own, but you should lance it and allow it to drain as it is very dangerous to have this pocket (abcess) burst internally and drain the poison into your bloodstream or lymph system.

Once you have lanced an abcess, it should be washed with one of the washes previously discussed, kept clean and regularly soaked in hot water as explained under puncture wounds. A drawing poultice can also be made from raw potato or any of the starchy root stalks listed in the plant chapter as having edible root tubers, such as cattail or yellow pond lily.

Another time-tested drawing poultice is made from fresh, clean powdered charcoal from your campfire (NOT ashes but the solid, black charcoal). Three of the best woods for this purpose are pine, spruce, and willow. The poultice is made by making a paste of the grated root or charcoal with water as hot as you can stand on your skin. This is held in place on the wound with a clean piece of cloth. As the poultice cools, replace it with more hot paste. This treatment also works very well on an abcessed tooth. If you are immersing a wound in a hot water soak, any of the above ingredients can be added to the water to increase the drawing capabilities.

If you find a wound becoming gangrenous, you definitely are in trouble. What is happening in this situation is the poison from the rotting dead tissue is gradually killing the healthy tissue next to it. If this situation is allowed to continue, the gangrene will keep working its way up the body until amputation of the limb is certain and death an imminent possibility. For this reason it is important to not ever allow an infection to get out of control. If for any reason a wound of any size begins to show signs of rotting tissue, ALL of this dead tissue must be removed immediately and the wound scrubbed thoroughly. After scrubbing, if antiseptic ointment etc. is not available, the wound must be washed with a strong decoction of alder bark or equisetum, followed by a charcoal poultice. Then the wound should be covered with a sterile dressing and bandage. If sterile dressings are not available, use as clean a cloth as is available.

A dressing should not be re-used as it is acting as poison collector and will recontaminate the wound. This applies to all wounds and burns. In a wilderness survival situation your medical supplies will be limited or nonexistant and your dressings may consist of parts of your T-shirt or other material. You may have no choice but to re-use them, even though this is against all standard medical practice. If you must re-use dressings, they must be washed as thoroughly as possible and then boiled for at least 15 minutes in clean water. The same should apply to any implements used in contact with the wound.

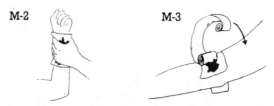

M-2   M-3

Section # 2—Controlling Bleeding

Hypovolemic shock, also called hemorhagic shock, is caused by loss of blood (from wounds) or plasma (as with severe burns). The greater the blood loss the greater the chance of shock. The sooner bleeding is stopped the better.

The preferred method is the use of direct pressure. This pressure is applied by pressing your hand over a sterile dressing directly over the wound. In most cases, severe bleeding can be controlled by this method. It is preferred to use a sterile dressing between the hand and the wound but if a sterile dressing is not available, use the cleanest piece of cloth you can find or if necessary, use just your hand. Using cloth or a gauze dressing will not only help keep the wound free of further contamination, but will absorb blood and help it clot (see figure # M-2).

A pressure bandage can also be used with success. A sterile gauze pad should be placed over the wound followed by a roll of gauze or a rolled bunch of gauze pads, all held tightly in place by a bandage tied firmly around the injuried limb (see figure # M-3). Elevation helps control bleeding by using gravity to lower the pressure of the blood at the injuried area. Elevation is used in combination with direct pressure and pressure dressings and in some cases can help greatly.

Blood is fed to all parts of the body through arteries. Pressure on the major artery feeding an injured area will reduce or stop the blood flow. This method should be used if direct pressure and elevation fail to stop bleeding from a wound. The specific spots on the body where an artery can be easily compressed against a bone are called pressure points (see figure # M-4). Do not use pressure points if direct pressure and elevation are working. When pressure points are used, all circulating in the limb is stopped. If pressure points are needed, by all means, use them.

The use of a tourniquet is always considered dangerous. If severe bleeding cannot be controlled by any other method, you will have no choice but to apply a tourniquet. The use of tourniquet as explained here is to stop the flow of blood to a wound and it will effectively accomplish this. Remember, it should only be used when the situation is life-threatening and direct pressure, elevation and pressure points have failed. Once a tourniquet has been applied, it should not be loosened. The loosening of a tourniquet can cause severe shock which can lead to death. This results from toxins built up in the injured limb while circulation is cut off by the tourniquet that are suddenly flooding to the heart when the tourniquet is loosened. Bear in mind that any time you apply a tourniquet, you must do so with the assumption that the limb will eventually be amputated.

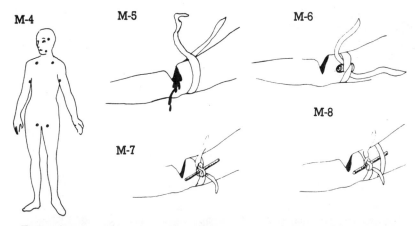

To apply a tourniquet you must find a spot between the heart and the wound, as close to the wound as possible without touching it. Place a rolled up piece of gauze or cloth over the main artery. Next, take another piece of material such as a cravat (triangular bandage) and place it around the injured limb and tie a half-hitch knot directly over the rolled gauze. A stick is then placed on the knot and a square knot tied over the stick (see figure # M-6 and M-7). The tourniquet is now tightened by twisting the stick just until the bleeding stops. Do not tighten beyond this point. Tape the stick securely in place (see figure # M-8). If the patient will soon be getting to a hospital or doctor, mark TK and the time the tourniquet was applied in an obvious place on the patient (like his forehead) to help the doctor make the proper assessment.

The tourniquet itself should be 1½ to 2 inches wide. Anything smaller will cut into the skin and injure subcutaneous tissue. A very effective tourniquet is a blood pressure cuff if you have one in your kit. It is gentle on the tissue under it and should be inflated only until the flow of blood is stopped. This is usually between 140 and 160 mm Hg on the gauge. A blood pressure cuff is a much safer tourniquet and can be safely inflated and left in place for up to 30 minutes without significant damage. There is another use for tourniquets applied in a different manner which will be explained later in this chapter.

Another method sometimes helpful in the control of bleeding is cryotherapy. This is simple the application of cold which reduces bleeding, swelling and pain by causing blood vessels to constrict. It is especially helpful to control subcutaneous bleeding in connection with sprains, dislocations or blows from blunt objects forceful enough to injure blood vessels well below the skin. In a winter survival situation there is usually plenty of ice and snow around to use for this therapy. Do not over-do it and freeze the injured area or you will have another whole set of problems. Figure # M-9 shows a safe method of using either ice or snow for this. If neither ice or snow are available, cloths soaked in very cold water will work.

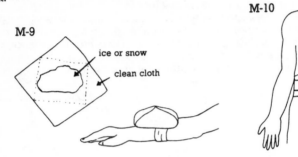

M-9

ice or snow

clean cloth

M-10

Many types of internal bleeding can also be controlled by a pressure dressing and bandage (see figure # M-10). The pressure will help to close off the ends of damaged blood vessels. Caution should be used if you feel there may be an underlying fracture in that area. In case of a fracture, too much pressure may cause additional damage to subcutaneous tissue.

Section # 3—Fractures and Dislocations

A fracture is any chip, crack or complete break of a bone. Fractures are classed into two major categories: open and closed. An open fracture is one that either the bone has come through the skin from the inside or a trauma from the outside has penetrated the skin and then broken the bone. In either case the fracture is considered to be open because the skin and subcutaneous tissue has been opened all the way to the broken bone.

A closed fracture is one in which the bone is broken but there is no opening of the skin and subcutaneous tissue associated with the fracture can be just as dangerous as an open fracture except for the possibility of contamination of the open wound.

Both open and closed fractures can be what are called angulated fractures. This simply means that the limb or joint has taken a new shape or unnatural position and in this case it is obvious that a bone or bones have been completely broken.

For first aid purposes, a fractured limb should be splinted in place (immobilized in exactly the position that you find it). This will prevent any further damage while the patient is being moved to a hospital. In the case of an open fracture, bleeding should be stopped and the open wound covered with a sterile dressing and bandage, and the limb splinted in place.

In a wilderness medical situation broken bones take on a whole new dimension. There is no doctor or hospital and you have to be mobile and able to work. You will have to be the doctor. Bear in mind that a broken bone can be a very serious injury an can cause damage to blood vessels, soft tissue and nerves. In the case of an open fracture, wound contamination can lead to very serious infection and permanent damage or loss of the limb. If you are with another person, it will make things much easier. If you are alone and injured, you will have to improvise ways of getting the job done. I will tell you what needs to be done but your situation will dictate how it is to be done.

If you feel you have a broken bone you must consider the signs and possible complications. If you felt the bone break or heard an audible snap, a bone is probably broken. If you try to move an injured limb and you hear a grating sound (called crepitus), you probably have a broken bone. Discoloration or swelling are symtoms of a fracture. Any major deformity indicates a broken bone or dislocated joint.

If you suspect a closed fracture, for example let's say it is the humerus (upper arm bone), your first move must be to check for pulse at the wrist (see figure # M-11). If there is no pulse, the ends of the broken bone are pinching off the flow of blood to your hand, which is carried there by the brachial artery. This is serious and circulation to the lower arm and hand must be restored or you face future amputation of the entire arm. Check next for skin temperature—if the hand or lower arm feels abnormally cold, there is usually a restriction of blood flow to that area.

M-11

radial pulse on
thumb side of
2 prominent tendons.

M-12

Check number three is for feeling and nerve response. Pinch or poke the skin of the hand for sensation. If there is no feeling, the hand is cold or there is no pulse, the fracture should be considered very serious. A fracture such as this should be tractioned and splinted with the traction left on if you are only hours or even a day away from medical help (see figure # M-12).

If you feel that it may be much longer than a day or two before rescue, the fractured bone or dislocated joint must be re-set. Almost always with this type of fracture, the amount of pain will immediately decrease once traction has been applied. In the survival situation, you should next gently feel the fracture area to check the alignment of the fracture and again feel for pulse and nerve response. At this point you should have both. If after tractioning, you have a pulse but only a partial nerve response, some of the nerves probably were damaged at the time of the fracture. Don't worry about this—there is nothing you can do. When you do get back to civilization, the fracture should be checked out by a doctor. Sometimes a neurologist can work wonders.

Now that the fracture has been tractioned and aligned, the traction should be released slowly, while checking for pulse and nerve response. If all goes well and the same pulse and nerve response remain, the fracture must now be splinted securely and not allowed to move until it is healed (see figure # 13). Note that the joint on either side of the fracture is immobilized.

M-13

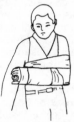

1) rigid splint with gauze roll in hand
2) support in sling
3) swathe across body to immobilize

If extreme discoloration is taking place in the area, there is probably some internal bleeding. If you feel that there are no bone chips, moderate pressure and elevation should control the bleeding. If you feel that there may be bone chips, the pressure point nearest the fracture should be used, along with elevation and cold packs. Stream water in much of the northern wilderness is 40° to 50° F and makes an excellent cold pack.

Next we will cover an open and angulated fracture, again using the humerus for our example. The distal (towards the extremity, away from the heart) end of the fractured bone is protruding through the skin in the superior (upper) lateral (outer) section of your arm. At the same time you notice your lower arm is twisted to an unnatural position. This is an open angulated fracture. There is obvious muscle damage, there is nerve damage and obvious blood loss. If bleeding is profuse it must be controlled first. If blood is pulsating or spurting from the wound, you have cut the brachial artery or one of its smaller branches. This is critical and your only concern at this point is to control the bleeding.

Once this has been accomplished, you must check for nerve response distally. In the upper arm close to the fractured humerus, are located the main nerves (the median, radial and ulnar) which controll all the motor functions of that arm. If you have a major loss of feeling or a problem with nerve response, at least one of these major nerves has been cut by the sharp ends of the broken bone, or hopefully is just being pinched between the pieces of bone.

Your next step is to irrigate the wound and the protruding end of the bone for the presence of any bone chips or foriegn material. These must be carefully removed. You must check thoroughly deep into the wound using sanitary procedure. Once the wound is free of any foreign material, you should again irrigate the wound and the area around it.

M-14

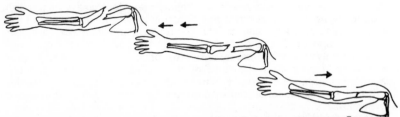

In this wilderness medical situation with no hope of outside medical help, you must traction, attempt to re-set the fracture and permanently close the

136

wound from outside contamination. This wound will require suturing which will be explained later. Figure # M-14 shows the tractioning and resetting procedure. Everything must be done slowly. You do not want to do any more damage than has already been done. After the limb has been tractioned, you must open the wound for final inspection and watch the bone ends align properly as you slowly release the traction. Splint the arm immediately but in such a way that you can easily get to and work on the wound.

During this process you should be checking distal pulse and nerve response. As with any bone or joint re-setting procedure, if there is no distal pulse or a decrease in nerve response, you must repeat the tractioning and re-setting procedure until there is satisfactory distal pulse. The wound will now need to be disinfected, sutured, covered with a sterile dressing and bandaged.

M-15a   M-15b

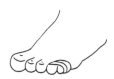

Any of the 206 bones in the human body can be broken but usual;y in wilderness accidents it is usually an arm or leg or their extremities. A broken toe should re-set and taped to the unbroken toe next to it. The broken toe wil act as a splint (see figure # M-15). A finger should be re-set and splinted with wood or something similar (see figure # M-16). There is little that can be done for a cracked rib, but a snug bandage may ease the pain. In any cervical (neck) injury, the neck must be tractioned and kept in traction until medical help is eventually secured (see figure # M-16).

M-16

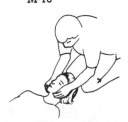

rolled towel or bulky
shirt to keep traction on
neck when manual traction
is released.

There is little I can tell you to do in a wilderness situation for a severe skull or spinal injury. I can advise you of some things NOT to do. Some signs of a head injury are:

    The injured person is unconscious
    The injured person shows a decreasing level of consciousness
    Any deformity, large swellings or depressions on the skull
    Any swelling behind the ear
    A deep laceration on the head
    A severe bruise on the head
    Unequal pupils
    Blackening color under the eyes
    Bleeding from the nose
    Bleeding from the ears
    Clear fluid coming from the nose or ears

137

Things NOT to do with a patient with a head injury:
Do not palpate (feel) the spot of injury
Do not probe the wound
For bleeding, do not apply direct pressure if bone fragments are present
For bleeding, do not apply direct pressure if there is a depression in the skull
For bleeding, do not apply direct pressure if a portion of the brain is exposed
Do not try to stop the flow of blood or clear fluid from the ears or nose
Do not remove any foreign objects protruding through the skull

Some signs of a spinal injury:
Pain in the back without movement
Deformity in the spinal column
Any spot along the spine is tender to the touch
Priapism (persistent erection of the penis)
Arms uncontrollably extended above the head
Loss of bladder or bowel control

Do's and Don'ts with a patient with a serious spinal injury:
Do NOT move the patient any more than absolutely necessary
Do keep the patient securely strapped to some sort of rigid back board if possible

A spinal injury is very serious—any movement can possibly cause permanent paralysis or death. In a wilderness survival situation not moving may mean freezing to death or dying of dehydration or starvation. What you do in this situation is a judgement call on your part. No author, survival instructor or doctor can make this decision for you.

A dislocation is that type of injury where a movable joint has been forced out of place. This can be serious at times. Soft tissue can be injured, along with blood vessels and nerves, and in some cases damage to the bone and joint capsule. In figure # M-17 you can see a typical movable joint and that same joint after it has been dislocated. The moment most dislocations occure, swelling will begin and in most cases the injury will be very painful. When a major joint such as a shoulder has been dislocated, you will not be able to use the arm connected to it.

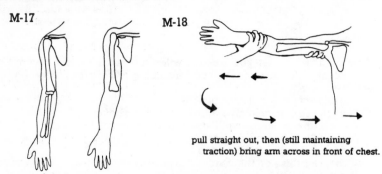

M-17 M-18

pull straight out, then (still maintaining
traction) bring arm across in front of chest.

The muscles attached near the joint will start to tighten up almost immediately. For these reasons, when in a wilderness medical situation, the joint must be re-set before the swelling and muscle spasms take over to such a degree that they fight you during the re-setting process. Also blood vessels and nerves may be pinched off at this point and this situation must be remedied as soon as possible. The two most important things to remember when re-setting a joint are: do it properly and do it as soon as possible.

In figure # M-18 you can see the proper method to re-set various joints. A basic rule of thumb is to traction the joint and then move the extremity attached to it in the direction that it would normally move. This should re-align the joint and take pressure off any blood vessels or nerves. You will now release traction. Check for nerve response. If you feel there is still a pinched nerve, repeat the procedure at once and then let it be. Remember there could have been a nerve injured at the time of the dislocation.

Immediately upon re-setting the pain should be reduced to almost nothing and swelling should be minimal if re-setting was done very soon after the injury occured. Application of cold packs will help reduce any pain and swelling that remains. In most cases, you will be able to use the extremity right away, if you are careful not to stress it too much. If possible, the extremity should be allowed to rest until fully healed. In the case of a shoulder, a sling should be employed if practical.

A good example to illustrate why fractures and dislocations should be re-set immediately is a fairly common injury sustained in vehicle accidents and falls where the ankle is dislocated, usually accompanied by a fracture, and causing the foot to fold inward. If not re-set within one hour there will be so much soft tissue damage that gangrene is almost inevitable even with hospital care. In the case of a completely broken femur (thigh bone), the powerful muscles that surround it will contract so much that the bone ends will be pulled drastically out of place. This also will happen within the first hour. To further complicate matters, a broken bone will start to mend itself within 3 hours, in whatever position it is left. All this means that delaying re-setting will make the procedure a great deal more difficult and painful and vastly increase the risk of permanently deforming the limb. Without hospital care, broken bones and dislocations must be re-set immediately—this is the opinion of a prominent Alaskan orthopedic surgeon.

Section # 4—Strains and Sprains

Both strains and sprains commonly occur in the wilderness. A strain is either the tearing or over-stretching of muscle. This can cause moderate discomfort to great pain when that muscle or group of muscles is used. Rest is the primary therapy. In the case of torn muscle, application of cold packs will ease the pain when the injury first happens. After that, rest and warm soaks will speed healing.

In the case of a sprain, the ligaments that connect bone to bone are damaged. This can be very painful and significant swelling may occur. Cold packs should be applied right after the injury occurs to help reduce swelling and pain. The sprained extremity should be rested and if possible, immobilized and treated like a fracture. This will promote healing and reduce pain. Warm soaks twice a day will help too.

Section# 5—Eye, Ear and Nose Injuries

As I've stated earlier, eye injuries can be very serious and that is why you shouldn't be walking around in the forest at night. If you do incur an eye injury, it should be attended to immediately. Your survival kit should include a signalling mirror which can now be used to help you see what is wrong with your eye. Many things can happen to your eyes, one of which is getting grit, sand or ashes blown into them. When this happens, do not rub them or you scratch the cornea. The cornea is the clear portion of the sclera which protects the pupil and iris and also helps focus light.

In most cases irrigating the eye will wash out any particles of dirt etc. Use clear water and as much as you need to do the job. Use your mirror to check that the eye has been washed completely clean. If the cornea has been scratched it will still hurt after the eye is clean and should be rested by keeping it closed and covered with an eye patch of some sort. The cornea will heal in one or two days.

Another common accident in the wilderness is getting a hot spark from your campfire in your eye. This should be treated the same as grit in your eye. The cornea will heal faster than any other tissue in your body but other than resting the injured eye, there is very little you can do for it medically.

A puncture wound to the eye is very serious. The entire posterior cavity is filled with a clear semi-liquid call vitreous humor which once lost, cannot be replaced. Neither the body nor the medical profession can restore it, so if the vitreous humor leaks out, the eye is lost permanently. If an object becomes impaled deeply into your eye, do not attempt to remove it. The injured eye must be covered with the impaled object left in place. Be very careful not to press or disturb the object. As soon as possible, see an opthamologist. Two very good washes for eye infections if you don't have opthalmic ointment are decoctions of alder bark or equisetum.

Another common eye injury in the north is snow blindness. When surrounded by unbroked snow or ice the eye can be subjected to too much sunlight and become sunburned. This is very painful and can leave you temporarily blind. In very bright sun on snow, a person can even become snow blind while wearing regular sunglasses. The best sunglasses for preventing snow blindness are "glacier goggles"—ones which have side panels to prevent refracted light from coming in around the lenses. Mirror lenses are most effective. You can improvise side panels out of many materials for your regular sunglasses.

M-19

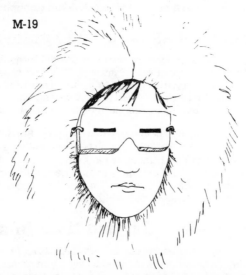

If you have no eye protection at all, you can improvise eskimo snow goggles out of wood, leather, cardboard, upholstery from an airplane seat or any heavy fabric. Cut narrow slits, just big enough to see out of and make sure they fit snugly across the bridge of your nose and around behind your eyes (see figure # M-19). Even a scarf tied around your face with narrow eye slits will help greatly. Make sure the slits are horizontal, not vertical, to allow you maximum lateral vision while minimizing reflected light.

If you do become snow blind or partially snow blind, wash your eyes with saline solution or the alder bark or equisetum washes, if available. Then you must prepare to shelter-in until your eyes heal. They must rest and be protected from all light. Depending on the severity of the burn, you may be totally blind for 2 to 4 days. Remember to use proper eye protection and avoid this injury.

In general, there are usually few inner ear injuries incurred in the wilderness. The most common ear injuries are to the pinna or auricle (outer ear). This is the part of the ear you can see and is made up of cartilage, skin and some soft tissue. It is subject to abrasions, lacerations, avulsions, burns and frostbite. There are some blood vessels and nerves in the pinna, but no major ones. Your concern will be stopping bleeding, sterilizing, closing the wound, if necessary, and applying a dressing and bandage. The general rules applying to these catagories of injuries also apply to the ear. If the ear has been crushed by a fall or a blow, always suspect possible brain damage. If blood or a clear fluid is draining from the inner ear, do not plug the ear or attempt to stop the flow. This is a sure sign of an injury to the brain and not the ear. You should never probe into the inner ear.

One common middle ear problem is an insect crawling deep into the ear canal. This is not a severe medical emergency, but a live insect trapped and buzzing deep inside your ear can drive you bonkers. You will have to get the insect out, but NOT by probing for it. The ideal remedy is to lie on your side, problem ear up, and fill the ear with sweet oil. You probably won't have that available to you so the next best thing will be to use warm (not hot) water and fill the ear until it overflows and the insect is gently flushed out.

The pain of an earache can often be helped by hot packs applied over the outer ear. If the ache is caused by an infection of the ear canal, a few drops of strong alder bark tea or a hot drawing poultice of charcoal or onion if available, will help. The ear can be flushed with hydrogen peroxide if there is an infection of the outer or middle ear. For an infection of the inner ear, rest and a diet high in vitamin C (from raw plants, especially willow leaves, spruce or pine needles or the new sprouts of any plant listed as having edible greens or stalks) and hot packs over the ear and the back of the neck are best treatment you will be able to come up with in a wilderness situation.

The two most common nose problems you might face are a simple nose bleed and a nosebleed caused by a fractured nose. Almost all simple nosebleeds can and should be controlled by your first finger and thumb. This should be done for approximately 10 minutes while in a sitting position with the nose elevated. If the nose continues to bleed, repeat the squeezing procedure and apply cold packs.

M-20

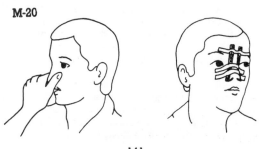

In the case of a fracture where the nose is displaced, it should be straightened and splinted (see figure # M-20). The nose will usually stop bleeding on its own after being re-aligned and splinted. Keep the head elevated for a short time and the nose and the bleeding should be OK. Application of cold packs will help stop bleeding, reduce swelling and ease the pain. If the upper part of the nose has driven or smashed into the face you should suspect possible brain damage. If this is the case check for other symptoms to be sure.

A congested nose or nasal passages can be relieved in the wilderness by several plants. Yarrow tea is excellent; eating or inhaling the vapors of cow parsnip or angelica (see plant chapter) will bring temporary clearing. In winter, you may find seeds on the dried stalks of cow parsnip sticking above the snow and use the vapors of boiling these seeds as a decongestant.

Section # 6—Shock

Everyone, I'm sure, has heard the term "shock" in relation to a medical trauma. There are many kinds of shock and for the most part, shock is the term used when the cardiovascular system fails to circulate adequate blood supply to all the parts of the body. In many cases shock can come on very slowly, but at other times it happens almost instantly. You must know the signs and symptoms of shock and what to do about it, as once it becomes deep shock, there is virtually nothing you can do to reverse it. As a rule of thumb, in any wilderness medical emergency, the patient should be treated for shock as a preventative measure.

Some of the different kinds of shock are:
* Cardiogenic shock—is commonly called heart shock. It results when the heart fails to pump an adequate supply of blood to each part of the body.
* Hemorrhagic shock—is commonly called bleeding shock or hypovolemic shock. It is caused by the loss of blood or plasma. Serious burns and wounds will lead to this type of shock.
* Neurogenic shock—is commonly called nerve shock. It results when the nervous system fails to control the changing diameter of the blood vessels. If the blood vessels become dialated and stay that way, there will not be enough blood pressure to fill these over-sized vessels and keep the circulation moving properly.
* Anaphylactic shock—is commonly called allergy shock. This is not uncommon in wilderness situations, so be aware of it. It can result from an insect sting or something you may eat or drink. You may have a severe allergy to something without being aware of it. Anaphylactic shock is always considered life-threatening.
* Metabolic shock—is commonly called body fluid shock. It is caused by the rapid and continued loss of body fluids through polyuria (excessive urination), diarrhea and vomiting. Dehydration, as talked about in an earlier chapter, can and will eventually lead to metabolic shock.
* Respiratory shock—is commonly called lung shock. It is caused by a decreased amount of oxygen in the blood and results from any serious lung injury.
* Psychogenic shock—is commonly called fainting shock. It is caused by fear or an adverse psychological reaction to the sight of blood or an injury. This results in the blood flow to the brain being neurologically interupted momentarily. The person then faints. This condition is temporary and the body will correct this problem shortly.

The signs and symptoms of shock are:
* weakness
* dizziness
* coolness
* thirst
* nausea
* feeling of fear
* cool, clammy skin sometimes accompanied by profuse sweating
* breathing becoming shallow and rapid
* pulse becoming rapid and weak
* cyanosis—skin, especially ear lobes and lips, becoming bluish
* Dilation of the pupils
* a drop in blood pressure. A drop of 5 points on the gauge is cause to be alert for shock. A pressure dropping to 90/60 in an adult is very serious and treating for shock must become an immediate priority.
* a lessening of awareness, responsiveness or coherant speech or thinking

Administration of oxygen is a definite life-saver in a medical situation where shock is present or a possibility. Unfortunately, in the wilderness, you probably won't have an oxygen unit. There are many compact oxygen units on the market and it's not a bad idea to stow one in your boat, aircraft or ATV. It could save a life someday.

As in any emergency, treatment for shock begins with ensuring that there is an adequate airway and that the injured person is breathing. If the person stops breathing, you will have to provide pulmonary resuscitation, and if both breathing and pulse have stopped, you will have to start CPR. If there is any bleeding it should be controlled. Any fractures should be corrected and splinted. Fractures will cause bleeding and pain which will aggravate a shock condition. Rough handling of the patient is also dangerous in a shock situation.

Keep the injured person lying still and warm. (A person in shock may need more blankets, etc. to keep warm than would a healthy person). If possible, make sure the injured person is not only covered on top, but also insulated underneath. You don't want to overheat the person either so monitor skin temperature continually. The patient must be kept warm and dry.

M-21

M-22

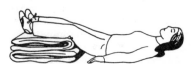 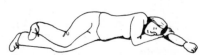

If there are no neck, spinal, serious head or chest injuries, the lower extremities should be elevated 12 to 18 inches (see figure # M-21). If breathing becomes difficult, the upper torso can be elevated. If the patient is unconscious, the position shown in figure # M-22 will allow the best drainage in the event of vomit or blood from internal injuries, etc. The supine position is used where there are major injuries to the extremities.

Remember, in all cases, monitor the injured person for any change in condition. Be alert for coronary or respiratory arrest and for vomiting. Vomiting can be very serious to an unconscious or very weak person. The victim may choke on his own vomit or aspirate it back into his lungs. In either case, the situation becomes life-threatening.

Section # 7
Circulatory and Respiratory Emergencies

In this section we will cover cardiopulmonary resuscitation (CPR), pulmonary resuscitation and opening airways. This is a very important subject that every man and woman in this country should be familiar with. Gretchen and I both teach this for the Red Cross, World Survival Institute and the Rural Education branch of the University of Alaska. I will cover the steps and procedures you must know, but I strongly advise everyone to take a CPR course from their local Red Cross or American Heart Association. It only takes 8 hours for the class but its value is beyond estimate.

As you know, breathing brings oxygen into our bodies and removes carbon dioxide, all the while maintaining the chemical balance of the blood. The instant a person's breathing stops and his heart ceases to beat, he is considered clinically dead. Within 4-6 minutes from that time, brain damage begins. 10 minutes after the heart has stopped there is significant brain cell death. This is called biological death and cannot be reversed. On the other hand, in many cases clinical death can be reversed.

M-23

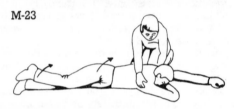

Part 1—Mouth-to Mouth Resuscitation. If a person is unconscious and seems not to be breathing, he must be rolled carefully as shown in figure # M-23, being careful to keep the body from twisting. Unless you know for sure to the contrary, assume the unconscious patient to have a possible cervical or spinal injury. If possible, just before rolling the person, gently feel along the spinal column and cervical area for any deformities in bone structure or alignment. If you feel a deformity, consider the person to have an injured vertebrae. If you move a person with such an injury, he might die or be permanently paralyzed. If on the other hand, you do not re-start the breathing, the victim will unquestionably die within a matter of minutes.

Next, you must open the airway and check for breathing. This is done by one of two accepted methods. The first is called the head tilt and has 3 variations: head-tilt, head-tilt chin-lift, and head-tilt neck-lift. Although these methods are excellent for opening the airway, they are not recommended for use on a victim with a cervical or spinal injury. The only widely recommended procedure for a person with a cervical or spinal injury is the modified jaw thrust.

M-24   M-25   M-26

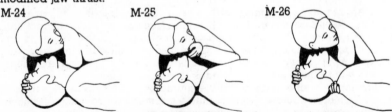

In figure # M-24 you can see the head-tilt maneuver. The procedure is a simple one. Place the palm and fingers of one of your hands on the victim's forehead and give firm, gentle backward pressure. This will tilt the head

144

backward and open the mouth and hopefully the airway. In figure # M-25 you can see the head-tilt chin-lift maneuver. This manuever will offer the maximum opening of the mouth and airway. One hand is placed on the forehead while the fingers of the other hand are positioned under the chin. The fingertips support the jaw and move the chin forward. Moderate pressure is exerted with the other hand on the victim's forehead.

In figure # M-26 you can see the head-tilt neck-lift technique. Place one hand on the victim's forehead and the other hand under the neck. As you lift the patient's neck, you push moderately down on the forehead. Be warned that the preceeding three maneuvers, while very effective for opening an airway, may severely aggravate a cervical or spinal injury, and so are not used where these injuries are suspected.

The modified jaw-thrust is the only procedure recommended for use on a victim with spinal or cervical injuries. In figure # M-27 you can see this technique. Rest your elbows on the ground as shown and place one hand on each side of the jaw. Following the contour of the jaw, push the jaw forward and apply most of the pressure with your index fingers. Whatever method you use, the airway must be opened. Once this has been accomplished, place your ear near the victim's mouth to feel and listen for breath, while you watch the victim's chest breathing movements. Spend 5 seconds on this check.

M-27   M-28

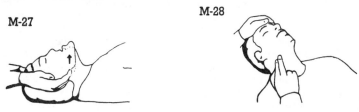

If the victim is not breathing, give 4 full breaths quickly. To accomplish this you must pinch the nose closed and blow directly into the person's mouth, making sure that your mouth is making a tight seal. These 4 breaths should be given fast enough that the lungs do not deflate between the breaths. Break the seal on the victim's mouth only long enough to get your next breath. Following this procedure, check the victim's pulse at the carotoid artery (see figure # M-28) while at the same time you look, listen and feel for breathing. This check should take no less than 5 seconds but no more than 10.

If the person is still not breathing but has a pulse, you must begin mouth-to-mouth breathing. Pinch the nose closed and take a deep breath. Make a seal over the victim's mouth. Blow the breath into the victim's mouth once every 5 seconds. If you don't have a watch, count after each breath, "one, one thousand, two, one thousand, three, one thousand, four, one thousand," breathe, "one, one thousand...." For practice, use a manniken or blow on a practice "victim's cheek. Never blow into the mouth of a person who is already breathing. You should blow into the victim's mouth about twelve timed breaths and then again check for a pulse and at the same time look, listen and feel to see if the patient has started breathing on his own. If there is still a pulse and no breathing, continue mouth-to-mouth breathing until he begins to breathe on his own.

Part 2 Mouth-to-Nose Resusitation. There may be a time when it may be impossible to give mouth-to-mouth resusitation. A victim may have severe lacerations to the lips, jaw or mouth or the jaws may be clamped shut so tight that you cannot open them. In these cases, open the airway by one of

145

the above methods, securely close and cover the victim's mouth with one hand and blow into the nose. Follow the same sequence as for mouth-to-mouth (see figure # M-29).

M-29

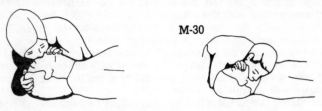

M-30

Part 3 Mouth-to-Stoma Resusitation. It is estimated that there are approximately 25,000 people in the U.S. that breathe through an opening in the front of the neck. This opening is called a stoma and is the result of an operation where all or part of the larynx has been removed. In a case such as this mouth-to-stoma resusitation is required. In some cases the person may still have an air passage from his lungs to the nose and mouth. If, when you blow into the stoma, the lungs do not inflate, you will have to cover the nose and mouth with hand (see figure # M-30). In some cases the victim may have a breathing tube inserted into the stoma. If the tube is plugged you will have to remove it with your fingers. Do not attempt to re-insert it. Again, follow the same procedure as for mouth-to-mouth resuscitation.

Part 4 Obstructed Airway. If, when attempting to fill the victim's lungs with air, you find that you cannot get any air in, re-position the head and try again. If this doesn't work, the victim may have an obstructed airway. It could be caused by anything from the victim's own tongue, vomit, food or an injury. If there is a visible object obstructing the airway, remove it. If you cannot see any obvious obstruction, the airway must be cleared following the techniques discussed in the section on choking.

M-31

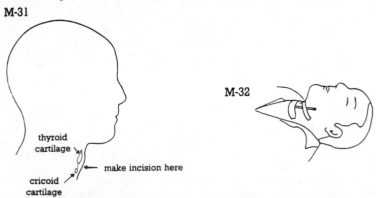

thyroid cartilage

make incision here

cricoid cartilage

M-32

Part 5 Cricothyrotomy. If ALL procedures to clear a totally obstructed airway fail, you will have to make an airway. If the victim does not start breathing, you have less than 10 minutes to rectify this life-threatening situation. Your only choice at this point is an operation called a cricothyrotomy. This operation is very simple but should be considered very dangerous.

The area around the Adam's apple should be sterilized, if possible, or at least cleaned very thoroughly. Alcohol, povidone (or some other form of iodine) or peroxide will work. You must now locate the cricothyroid mem-

146

brane located between the Adam's apple (thyroid cartilage) and the cricoid cartilage with your fingertips (see figure # M-31). Once you are sure of the location, make a vertical incision straight through the membrane. This incision will have to be kept open or it will collapse. Any small hollow tube will serve, from a ballpoint pen without its filler to a rifle cartridge with bullet, powder and primer removed. Once the improvised cannula (which was sterilized or at least very thoroughly cleaned before insertion) is in place in the incision and working, it should be taped in position (see figure # M-32).

If you have assembled a proper survival and medical kit, you will have very servicable plastic tubing for this application. If and when the original obstruction is removed, the cannula can be removed and the area re-sanitized and closed with a butterfly. This incision will heal in a short time if properly taken care of. Like all wounds it should be covered with a sterile dressing until it is healed. WARNING: This is to be considered a serious operation and can have complications such as accidentally cutting the recurrant laryngeal nerve which would affect the voice; the esophogus or even the upper part of a lung might be cut. Be sure of your location before making the incision.

Part 6 Cardiopulmonary Resuscitation (CPR). As we covered pulmonary resuscitation we were concerned only with the victim's breathing. The heart was still working because we could feel a pulse. The heart can continue beating for a limited amount of time even though the breathing has completely stopped. Because of this, only pulmonary resuscitation was needed. If for any reason the heart fails to function (cardiac arrest), the lungs will also stop working (respiratory arrest). At this point, the victim needs CPR. Not only will you have to breathe for the person, but you will also do chest compressions to force the heart to circulate the oxygen-enriched blood throughout the body. This can in many cases, start the heart beating again on its own.

The reason chest compressions work is the heart is being squeezed between the sternum (breastbone) and the backbone. As you release the compression, the heart returns to its original shape and ready for the next compression. The heart is simply a pump and by giving proper chest compressions you are making the heart continue to circulate the blood throughout the body. By breathing properly into the victim's mouth, nose or stoma you are forcing the lungs to exchange carbon dioxide for oxygen. If done correctly, you are, for all intents and purposes, keeping the person alive.

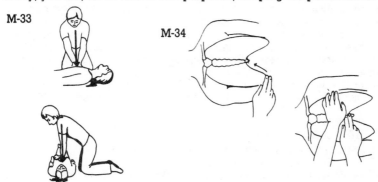

M-33

M-34

Part 7 One-Person CPR (Adult). CPR can be given by either one or two people. In this part we will discuss one-person CPR. Once you have ascertained that the victim is neither breathing nor has a pulse, (look, listen and feel for breathing, while feeling for a pulse in the carotoid artery), CPR must begin. As explained in the section on pulmonary resuscitation, the victim must be rolled carefully over onto his stomach. You must now position yourself as shown in figure # M-33. Locate the xyphoid process by tracing the edge of the ribs with your index and middle fingers until you find the notch at the very center of the lower chest. This is the point where the ribs meet the bottom of the sternum. Keeping your index finger on this spot, measure up two finger widths from the notch (see figure # M-34). Now place the heel of your other hand just above and touching your fingers which are measuring up from the xyphoid. The heel of your hand should now be directly over the victim's heart.

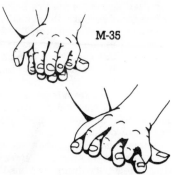

M-35

If you accidentally give compressions over the xyphoid process, there is a good chance of injuring the liver. Make sure you are not giving compressions too low on the chest. Once the heel of your first hand is in proper position, your other hand must be placed over it. The fingers can be laced together or left straight out, just so they do not make contact with the victim's chest—only the heel of your first hand should be touching (see figure # M-35). You will need power to give proper compressions but you must also be comfortable as you may be doing it for quite some time and will need all your strength. You must be kneeling, not sitting on your heels and your shoulders should be directly over the victim's sternum so you can push straight down on the heart. As you find a position giving you both comfort and strength, always be aware of proper hand placement—two fingers above the xyphoid and fingers not touching the chest (a proper compression would give enough force to those improperly placed fingers to fracture ribs). As you push down, you should be compressing the victim's chest a full 4 centimeters (1½ to 2 inches). Your movements should all be smooth, strong and rythmic, never jerky. As you are coming back up from a compression, maintain hand contact so that you do not loose your location on the chest.

When performing one-man CPR the compressions should be given at the rate of 80 compressions per minute. It helps to count out loud, saying, "one-and two-and three-and four-and..." Remember that while you are giving CPR the victim must always be lying on his back on a firm surface. The victim's head should be level with or slightly lower than the body to ensure adequate blood flow to the brain. The feet may be slightly elevated. Do not interupt CPR to elevate the lower body. Timing is critical and proper compressions and breaths are important. The sequence for one-man CPR is as follows:

* check for consciousness
* establish and open airway
* look, listen and feel for breathing
* give 4 rapid breaths
* check for pulse (while you look, listen and feel for breaths)
* locate the compression spot
* form proper hand position
* begin compressions—set of 15 compressions, then:
* 2 quick breaths after each set of 15 compressions
* after 4 complete sets of 15 compressions, 2 breaths, check for pulse and breathing for at least 5 seconds

148

CPR must be continued until the victim's heart starts beating on its own and ventilations continued until the victim is breathing on his own or you are physically unable to continue because of exhaustion. Practice CPR on a manniken. If you use a live person to practice, do not ever actually make compressions or you may disrupt their normal heart rhythm.

Part 8 Two-Person CPR. Two person CPR follows the same general rules as one-person with the following changes:

* 2 rescuers work on one victim
* one person ventilates at the rate of one breath every 5 compressions
* the second person gives compressions at the rate of 60 per minute, counting, "one-one thousand, two-one thousand, three-one thous- and, four-one thousand, five-one thousand, one-one thousand, two- one thousand...." continuing steadily without interuption
* Every one or two minutes, the person ventilating must tell the person giving compressions to stop for a pulse check. The ventilator will check for pulse for a few compressions while the compressor is still giving compressions to be sure that the compressions are creating adequate circulation, then will say "Stop for pulse check" and check for pulse and look, listen and feel for breathing. If there is no pulse, the ventilator gives a full breath and says, "continue compressions". If there is a pulse but no breathing, the ventilator will say, "We have a pulse" and continue ventilating at one breath every 5 seconds. If there is both pulse and breathing, both rescuers will continue with whatever treatment the victim requires, all the while, monitoring pulse and breathing frequently.
* The person giving ventilations must time himself to the compressor's count. Under no circumstances should the compressor change his rhythm or hestitate for the ventilations. The ventilator should take in a deep breath on the count of four and blow into the victim exactly at the end of the 5th compression just when the chest is beginning to rise.
* When the compressor becomes tired, he may call to change places, saying, "change, one-thousand, two-one thousand..." As he gives his fifth compression, the ventilator will give one more breath and move into position to begin compressions and with his fingers, locate the compression spot. The second rescuer, meanwhile has begun a 5 second pulse and breathing check. If there is no pulse or breathing, the new ventilator gives a breath and says, "Begin com- pressions" and the sequence continues as before.

Part 9 Choking Victim. Many people die each year from choking. In most cases it is because of food lodged in their throats. In the wilderness this can easily happen. You may procure a type of meat that is extremely tough and you may try to swallow it without chewing it. It becomes lodged in your throat and your airway is now closed. By now we all know how serious a closed airway is. If the situation is not immediately corrected, death is immi- nent. If this his happening to someone else in your party ask him if he can speak. A person with a completely closed airway cannot speak, cough or breathe. If the airway is almost completely blocked, he will not be able to forcibly cough, he will have extreme difficulty breathing, and you may notice high-pitched noises each time he tries to inhale. This person should be treated as though his airway is completely closed, as this situation is also life-threatening.

If, however, a person can speak and is coughing forcefully, he should be left alone. Forceful coughing is the most effective method to clear an obstructed airway. If the victim cannot speak, you must immediately rectify the problem or your conscious choking friend will soon become unconscious and shortly thereafter, dead. Hold the victim as shown in figure # M-36, supporting the person with one hand on his chest, keeping the victim's head lower than his chest. Strike the person over the spine between the shoulder blades (see figure # M-36). Four blows should be delivered quickly and forcefully with the heel of your hand. You are attempting to loosen the obstruction and not break the victim's back. Use common sense.

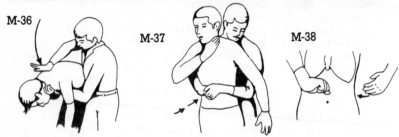

If the 4 back blows do not clear the airway, you must next give 4 abdominal thrusts. Change your position to that shown in figure # M-37. Locate the navel and the xyphoid process (put your little finger on the navel and your thumb on the xyphoid). Make a fist with your other hand and place it, thumb inwards, against a spot midway between the navel and xyphoid. Now place you first hand over the second (see figure # M-38). If you place your hands to high you will damage the liver (which will cause the victim to bleed to death internally) and if you place them too low, you will be ineffective. Now pull inwards and upwards forcefully. Repeat this 4 times. If the airway does not clear, go back to 4 back blows. Repeat this until the airway is clear or the victim loses consciousness.

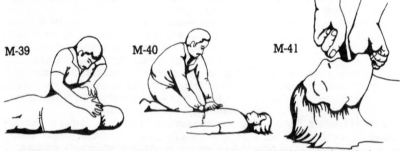

If the victim loses consciousness, position yourself and the victim as shown in figure # M-39. Give 4 back blows. If not successful roll the victim towards you onto his back and give 4 abdominal thrusts as shown in figure # M-40, again locating the spot midway between the navel and the xyphoid. This time however, you will be using the heel of your hand rather than your thumb. The thrust is still inward and upward.

After the 4 abdominal thrusts, grasp the person's lower jaw and tongue and pull the jaw out and upward to open the mouth (see figure # M-41). With the index finger of your other hand, sweep across the mouth deep down to the base of the tongue. Do not probe straight in or the obstruction may be pushed deeper into the airway. After you have swept the mouth, tip the head as shown in the CPR section. Check for breathing. If there is none, try to give 4 quick breaths. If the lungs will not inflate, repeat the sequene of 4 back blows, 4 abdominal thrusts, mouth sweep, check for breathing, 4 quick breaths. If there is no breathing but you can inflate the lungs, after the

4 quick breaths, check for pulse. If there is pulse, begin mouth-to-mouth resuscitation. If there is neither pulse nor breathing, but you can inflate the lungs, begin CPR. If the lungs do not inflate keep up the above sequence until the airway is cleared.

If you come upon a person that is already unconscious and is not breathing, try to give 4 quick breaths. If the lungs will not inflate, consider the airway blocked and begin the procedure outlined for the choking victim who has become unconscious.

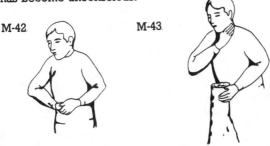

M-42   M-43

If you are alone and have a fully obstructed airway, you must act quickly. Give yourself abdominal thrusts as shown in figure # M-42 or by using a rock, stump, etc. as shown in figure # M-43. Be careful that in your haste you locate the proper spot between the navel and the xyphoid. You can very easily lacerate your own liver by delivering these thrusts too high. Continue these thrusts until you clear the airway.

Section # 8—Hypothermia

Hypothermia is a very serious medical problem that can easily become life-threatening. Hypothermia is the cooling of the body below its normal temperature of 97° to 100° F. The human body must remain within this range or complications will begin. If the temperature of the body is allowed to drop too far, coma and death result. This is a common wilderness problem and a very deadly one. In the first stages of hypothermia, the cappillaries at the skin surface begin to constrict. Your body does this automatically to minimize heat loss and keep the internal (core temperature) of your body warm even at the expense of outer tissues. When this begins, you will start to shiver—the first sign that you are becoming hypothermic.

As the situation progresses, the body core temperature begins to drop. A drop in core temperature to 96°, a mere 2° change, will cause uncontrollable shivering. You will not be able to accurately control your hands and fingertips. It will become difficult to perform chores like building a fire to keep warm. Your mind is still functioning but this uncontrollable shivering is your last warning before hypothermia begins to affect your power of judgement. You are at this point, in serious trouble and must do something about it. When the core temperature gets down to 90° to 95°, shivering will become so violent that you will have trouble speaking and at that point, your decision-making ability will be impaired.

At core temperatures of 86° to 90° shivering will diminish, your skin will take on a bluish color and/or become puffy. Muscle control will be very poor and you will not be able to make a rational decision. Your posture will become poor and your muscles rigid. If the core temperature continues to drop, between 81° and 85° you will become totally irrational, your pulse and respiration will slow down. If the core temperature is further reduced to 78° to 80° you will become unconscious, your heartbeat erratic and your

151

reflexes cease to function. Below 78° you will have a coronary and pulmonary arrest and in ten minutes will be dead.

As you can see, hypothermia is no joke. It kills people who ignore its early signs. People who are too "tough" to worry about shivering become statistics. The best treatment is to prevent it—keep warm. Don't be macho and under-dress. When hypothermia conditions exist there are no macho people, only cautious ones and dead ones.

Hypothermia often results from an accident over which you had no control like an overturned boat or a sudden drop in outside temperature you weren't expecting. You must always be on the watch for hypothermia warning signs and symptoms, which include simple shivering, drowsiness, numbness and apathy at first. Even in the early stages of hypothermia you will have the inclination to do things the easy way even if you know that it's the wrong way. Next, the shivering will become uncontrollable and your mental capabilities will decrease. Speech may be slurred, eyesight may begin to fail, breathing and pulse will slow down. This is followed shortly by unconsciousness and death. Don't forget about the shivering slowing down or stopping—this is a critical warning. Memorize and be able to recognize the signs. They are the key to survival if hypothermia starts.

Treatment for hypothermia is heat. If you start to become hypothermic or you recognize the signs in someone with you, stop what you are doing and get warm. I don't mean an hour from now. You may not have an hour. Put on more clothes, get out of the wind, build a fire, get dry, heat water and drink it, if available, eat sugar or candy. Do not drink alsohol, it will make you feel warm temporarily but will actually dilate your capillaries so that crucial core heat will be lost to the outside air. Remember, most hypothermia deaths occur when the outside temperature is between 30° and 50° above zero F.

If you come across a person that is severly hypothermic, he must be warmed. Ideally he should be immersed in 110° water, clothes and all. In the wilderness, this probably will not be possible, but you can make the victim some sort of shelter from the wild, remove wet clothing and replace with dry if possible. If you have a sleeping bag, remove wet clothes and put him in it. Place leak-proof water bottles of very warm water or warm rocks (not hot enough to be uncomfortable to your skin) near his throat, armpits and groin. Build a warm fire to radiate heat to him. If he is conscious, give him warm, non-alcoholic drinks, ones which contain sugar if possible. Watch him closely, he may go into cardiac arrest as the pooled blood in his extremities reach his heart. You may need to perform CPR after you start rewarming a hypothermia victim.

Section # 9—Frostbite

Frostbite is broken down into 3 categories of degree—frostnip, superficial frostbite and deep frostbite. Frostbite can be an extremely serious problem. Anytime the tissue of the body freezes, it is a severe trauma to that part of the body. Frostbite can cause the loss of toes, fingers, arms, legs or life itself. Although this book is concerned with wilderness survival, frostbite is a problem in cities and towns. Preparedness and prevention are the answer but if it does happen correct treatment can prevent amputation.

As a wilderness survivor, you must know how to prevent, recognize and treat frostbite. I live in an area where it is not uncommon for winter temperatures to plunge to 70° or even 80° below zero F and stay that way for days. A normal winter day is 40° to 50° below zero. I respect the cold and I've seen it kill. I spend most of my days outdoors and teach arctic survival in the middle of winter. I've never had a student get frostbite and I have never frostbitten so much as a finger on my hand or the nose on my face. The point I am making here is not that I am very tough—that has nothing to do with wilderness survival—but that I am extremely cautious. Just one mistake at 70° below and you are in trouble. So remember, prevention in the best cure.

There are several factors to consider in preventing frostbite. The first is knowing your environment: how the weather acts and what is the worst you can expect. Know what is possible and prepare for the worst. By being prepared I mean really thinking about it and outfitting yourself accordingly. I'll give you my system and use myself as an example. Let's say I'm going out for a week on the trapline. The first thing I do is tell Gretchen or someone exactly where I'm going and how long I intend to be gone. This is important if something goes wrong. A good example of something going wrong would be rolling my snowmachine and breaking a leg. The snow machine could be damaged and won't run. It's 50° below and a long cold spell is setting in to stay a while.

I only have three things going for me at this point. I'm prepared for the worst which is happening like a fast run movie all around me, my knowledge of wilderness and medical skills, and the fact that I told Gretchen that I'd be back in exactly one week. Not eight or nine days but exactly seven and I know that by 12 midnight on the seventh day she will be on her way to help me.

Let's say that in the snow machine accident I lost my fur hat. In this case it's not a catastrophe because I always stuff a wool watch cap in my parka pocket. To be without head protection at extreme low temperatures is real trouble. I have on layered clothing and because of the pain in my leg I am beginning to perspire. As I remove my parka, I notice a 12 inch tear in the back. In this case my parka is filled with thinsulite and thank God, not down. If it were down the countryside would be covered with tiny goose feathers and I would have a useless parka. Down parkas are pretty and light but don't belong in the wilderness. I am now ready to attend to my injury and because my survival and medical kits are properly assembled, this in no problem. Next I will build a fire, start my water generator and make a shelter. In this situation I will be fine, but only because I anticipated the worst and safeguarded against hypothermia, frostbite and dehydration.

Some factors that lead to frostbite are:
* inadequate clothing
* fatigue
* too much alcohol
* restricted circulation (boots or clothing too tight)
* long exposure
* low temperature, especially combined with wind

Frostnip is the least serious form of frostbite and commonly happens to the tip of the nose, ears, fingers and toes. The skin turns white and the condition is usually painless. It is a warning however, and can progress to more serious frostbite.

Superficial frostbite usually happens to the fingers, hands, toes, feet and face. Sometimes knees and upper legs are frostbitten by wearing light pants with no long underwear in cold, windy conditions. The tissue will look white, waxy and firm. The area will be numb and may have a blue or purple outline.

Deep frostbite is complete freezing of a portion of the body. The affected area will be white and hard. It will be painless and completely numb while frozen.

Treatment: Frostnip may be thawed as soon as it occures by covering the affected area. All other frostbite should NEVER be thawed if there is a chance of re-freezing it. It is much better to walk miles on a frozen foot than to thaw it and later have it re-freeze while you are walking. If it is re-frozen the damage to the tissue will be compounded and you will very likely later face amputation. When you are in a secure situation and can safely thaw the affected part, always use a gentle soak in water that is kept at a temperature of 100° to 110° F. If you have no thermometer, a rule of thumb is that the water should feel quite warm but not uncomfortable to your wrist or some non-frozen part of your body. The water must be maintained at this temperature for as long as the thawing process takes, which may be up to ½ hour.

Watch for all the white flesh to turn pink or red. At this point you will experience extreme pain. Large blisters called blebs will form within a day. Do not break them. They are a good sign and if left intact, will guard against infection. Before the blebs form you should separate frozen toes from each other by placing sterile gauze, or the cleanest material you have available, between them. The same applies to fingers or ears or any place that damaged tissue lies against other flesh. Blebs will break on their own, usually in 2 or 3 weeks. When they do, be extremely careful of contamination and infection. Use an antiseptic ointment. Treat the area like a burn (see following section). In the case of deep frostbite, a hard, black carapace will form over the area. Do not remove it—it is protecting damaged tissue while it heals. This carapace will sluff off on its own in 3 to 6 weeks. If all goes well, and you guard against infection, the area will heal itself within 6 months to a year.

If all does not go well the area will become foul and eventualy gangrenous with the possibility of blood poisoning. In this case you must treat the area as described for a wound that is becoming gangrenous (see section on wounds). The do nots of frostbite treatment are: do not rub the area to thaw it, especially with snow. The tissue is very fragile at this point. Do not thaw slowly in cold water. Do not thaw by holding close to a fire. This may sound obvious, but remember a frozen limb has no feeling while frozen and too many people have charred a frozen limb and not realized it until they smelled the burning flesh. Frostbite is dangerous; respect the cold, be cautious and prepared for the worst climactic conditions possible and don't let yourself get into this situation.

Section #10—Burns

Burns are another medical problem that often happens in the wilderness. Depending on the degree, burns range from merely uncomfortable to life-threatening. All burns that open the skin are very susceptible to infection. You MUST do everything possible to keep a burned area sterile. Burns are classed into 3 categories. A first degree burn is one that involves only the epidermis (first layer of skin). The skin will appear red and possibly show some sign of swelling. This burn will heal on its own and is not considered serious. It can be painful but certainly not life-threatening.

A second degree burn is serious. This burn has destroyed the epidermis and damaged the dermis (the second layer of skin). Subcutaneous has not been damaged but is now exposed to contamination. This situation provides a good media for infection so be aware of this possible problem and treat it accordingly. Mild cases of second degree burns will again heal themselves when treated with a certain amount of care. Second degree burns will be very red, blisters will appear and what's left of the skin will appear spotted. There will be intense pain and swelling for about 48 hours from the time of injury. In more severe cases of second degree burns there will be more fluid loss. Fluid loss is the second threat from severe burns and can be just as deadly as infection. Usually with second degree burns, fluid loss is not severe but be very careful to prevent infection.

A third degree burn is very serious and at times can be hard to distinguish from a severe second degree burn. A third degree burn has not only destroyed the first two layers of skin, but has damaged deeper tissues. This burn will have severe fluid loss and be extremely prone to infection. This is called a full-thickness burn and trauma to the affected area is major. A third degree burn is recognized by certain areas sometimes being charred black and areas that are hard and white. Extreme pain may be experienced from areas surrounding the completely destroyed tissue. The greater the surface area burned, the greater the fluid loss and the greater the risk of infection. Immediately following a burn injury, the area should be flooded or immersed in clean, cold water to cool it and stop the progression of tissue damage and pain.

In a first-aid situation, the burn should be covered with a sterile dressing and the patient transported to the nearest emergency facility. In a wilderness emergency, the burn should be thoroughly irrigated with sterile cool water, or the cleanest water available. All debris, gravel, wood, bits of burned clothing, etc., must be removed. If you have a properly assembled medical kit, now is the time you will really need it. Once the burn has been irrigated and cleaned, it should be irrigated with peroxide followed by a light coating of some form of iodine. Then the burn should be coated with an antibiotic ointment. At this point I would cover it with a non-adhering (adaptic) regular sterile gauze pad if you have no non-adhering dressings, but never use an occlusive (air-tight) dressing.

The dressing must be removed EVERY day and the wound scrubbed with a sterile gauze pad and peroxide. This daily regimen is VERY IMPORTANT and ALL white or yellow dead tissue and crust MUST BE REMOVED EVERY DAY. The scrubbing and removal of dead tissue will make the burn bleed a little and this is a very good sign. Scrubbing will be very painful but under no circumstances should the burn be allowed to scab over. Scabs, yellow crust and dead tissue is a perfect breeding ground for bacteria. Keep this process up and the burn will heal from the inside out with no infection. After scrubbing, clean the area with an iodine solution, coat with antibiotic ointment and cover with a new sterile dressing and bandage. If you are using non-adhering dressings they will come off easier when you change dressings than will regular gauze pads. This process must be continued until the burn has healed over with healthy, pink skin. As discussed in the section on wounds, it is understood that you may find yourself without sterile dressings. If so, follow the same procedures to sterilize makeshift dressings. Just remember that with burns, even more than any other injury, infection is a very likely and deadly possibility.

Now that you know how to safeguard against infection, you must understand the why's and hows of fluid replacement. With a severe burn, fluid loss is a serious complication and this fluid must be replaced right away. IV's (intravenous solutions) of ringers lactate and D5W for the first day are the ideal treatment followed by plasma replacement. Unfortunately, you probably will not have these with you in the wilderness so I won't elaborate. My large kit contains IV solutions and IV apparatus and whenever possible, it goes with me, at least as far as base camp. You probably will not have enough sterile dressings, antibiotic ointments and antiseptic irrigation solutions so you will be improvising as described in the section on wounds. Irrigation will be done with boiled, cooled water and alder bark and equisetum decoctions will be your antiseptics. Cleaned and boiled pieces of cloth will be your sterile dressings. Even though you are improvising, follow sanitary procedures and think infection prevention.

To improvise on fluid replacement, you will have to administer fluids orally. The amount of water needed will vary according to the size of the burned area, but as a rule of thumb, be planning to administer 5 or more quarts of water in the first 8 hours and another 5 quarts over the next 16 hours. You will have to monitor the flow of urine and if it becomes extremely high, start cutting back on the water. If urine flow is low, increase the amount of water. If the patient begins to vomit from too much water, you will have to cut back. But you should administer as much fluid as the patient can tolerate. As previously discussed under dehydration, you must be very conscious of maintaining the electrolye balance when consuming massive amounts of plain water. Follow the plan listed under the section on dehydration in the chapter on water. Always, when dealing with severe or extensive 2nd degree and all 3rd degree burns, be prepared for and treat for shock.

Section # 11
Miscelaneous Conditions and Treatment

Part 1 High Altitude Sickness. This sickness can be divided into 3 separate conditions. The first is high altitude pulmonary edema. This condition usually strikes at altitudes above 8,000 feet and usually to people between ages 5 and 18, but all ages may be susceptible. Symptoms come on gradually over the course of several days. These symptoms include headaches, coughing, shortness of breath and a general feeling of weakness. As the condition progresses the pulse rate will increase, accompanied by a low fever. Congestion in the chest will become obvious along with bloody sputum. As with all high altitude sicknesses, descent to lower altitude is the primary treatment. This should be done immediately. If oxygen is available, use it. Tourniquets can be used in a different way than the normal application. Three tourniquets should be placed on three of your limbs, tightened only to the point of slightly restricting, not stopping the flow of blood. Every five minutes, take one tourniquet off and put it on the free limb. Rotate every five minutes until you arrive at lower altitude where symptoms begin to diminish. Pulmonary edema is fatal if not treated promptly.

Acute mountain sickness is the second high altitude disease. It usually strikes at 10,000 feet or above. The symptoms are very similar to pulmonary edema with the addition of vomiting. The treatment is again, immediate descent. If vomiting is severe, the patient will need fluid replacement and oxygen if available.

Cerebral edema is the most dangerous of the three altitude conditions. It can happen as low as 8,000 feet. Beginning symptoms may be similar to the other two but as it progresses, the victim will become mentally and emotionally unstable and will start to show serious signs of neurological disorder with vision, walking and paralysis of certain muscles, especially the facial muscles. At this point, the victim is very close to becoming comatose and death will follow shortly. Again, the most important treatment is immediate descent and oxygen if possible.

It may be hard to tell one form of altitude sickness from the others, and it may not be very important to do so. What is important is that you recognize all the symptoms and if a person is experiencing any one symptom or especially two or more, that the victim is immediately removed to lower altitude and treated with oxygen if it is available. Altitude sickness is only serious if you allow it to become so.

Part 2 Nausea and Vomiting. In a wilderness survival situation, vomiting may or may not be considered life-threatening. It may be caused by something you have eaten or an internal infection or various other factors. In

156

the case of spoiled or disagreeable food, vomiting will clear the stomach of the offending food. If however, vomiting continues for more than 5 minutes or so, I would consider the condition serious, with the possibility of leading to a dangerous dehydration condition. Treatment in a wilderness situation consists of administering powdered charcoal from your campfire in water. Mix at least 1 tablespoonful in a half a cup of water and drink it. Follow with a cup or two of tea made with raspberry leaves or yarrow (see plant chapter) to soothe the stomach. Nausea can sometimes be alleviated (and thereby prevent vomiting) by applying hot packs (cloths soaked in hot water and covered with something to prevent cooling. Temperature should be as hot as is comfortable.) to the abdomen.

Part 3 Food Poisoning. Food poisoning can easily happen if you are not careful in the wilderness. But then again, every year people get sick and sometimes die from commercially packaged food off the grocers' shelves. When I read the ingredients on the labels of many "U.S.D.A. inspected" packages and containers, I sometimes wonder how anyone can survive after eating it. At any rate, if while eating or immediately after eating, you feel sick and the possibility exists that you have been food poisoned, do not wait until you become sicker. Induce vomiting immediately and you may get rid of most of the poison before your body absorbs it all. In my large kit I keep a commercial poison antidote kit and you would be wise to do the same. The antidote kit contains two vials, one of which is an emetic (a substance that will induce vomiting) called syrup of ipecac and the other is simply a solution of powdered charcoal, a purifier.

Incidently, ipecac is only the powdered roots of a tropical plant and charcoal is merely burned wood. Amazing! This antidote kit which is carried on board the most modern ambulances is a simple, old-fashioned natural remedy. Nature is still supplying the remedies, just not getting credit for it. Vomiting is nature's stomach pump and in the case of food poisoning will do the best job. For poisoning in general, if the poison you have ingested is a petroleum product, strong acid or strong alkali (caustic), DO NOT induce vomiting.

The most common form of poisoning you are likely to encounter in the wilderness will be food poisoning from spoiled meat or fish or mistakenly eating a poisonous plant. Immediate vomiting can be induced by drinking the syrup of ipecac from your antidote kit, or if you don't have it, by drinking 3 or 4 cups of salt water quickly and then if you haven't already vomited, put your fingers as far back in the throat as necessary to bring on the desired response. Once your stomach has been thoroughly emptied, you should feel an immediate relief, but you should now do something to soothe your stomach and absorb any remaining poison. Take the charcoal preparation in your antidote kit, or make up a preparation of water and powdered charcoal from your campfire. Follow this with a cup of tea made from raspberry leaves, yarrow, wild rose petals or fireweed blossoms. Food poisoning is more than unpleasant, it can be life-threatening and can cause severe diarrhea that will bring on dehydration and exhaustion. Treat it immediately if you suspect it. When eating wild plants for the first time or questionable meat, follow the testing procedure outlined in the plant chapter.

Part 4 Appendicitis. Appendicitis can be a very serious wilderness medical problem and since you didn't expect it, you won't have a pharmacy with you. This condition is life-threatening if the appendix bursts and the ideal answer is immediate evacuation and surgery. If you must take care of it yourself, you must properly recognize it. In a properly planned medical kit will be two thermometers—one for normal use and one for hypothermia (one that will read to very low temperatures). The appendicitis patient will probably have a temperature of between 99° and 101°. The patient will usually feel minor pain around the area of the navel at first. After the first few hours the pain will move to the lower right quadrant of the abdomen (see figure # 44). This shift in location of the pain is very important.

M-44

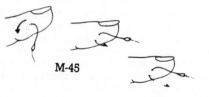

pain moves from the navel to lower-right quadrant.

The patient will experience pain if the area is touched. If all these symptoms are present, consider the condition appendicitis and life-threatening. Another technique used in diagnosis is to touch the area opposite the site of the pain with more pressure and then remove the hand quickly. If pain is then experienced in the area of the appendix shortly thereafter, the appendicitis is probably well advanced. Treatment without proper medical facilities and personnel, is as follows. If the condition has advanced to the point where the victim has taken a fetal position, cover him and keep him warm and resting. Alternate hot and cold packs applied to the location of the pain may help. Watch for signs of shock and treat for it.

The patient will, in most cases, recover in two or three weeks, although he will still experience considerable discomfort. The critical period will be the first three days. During the entire time that the condition exists and well as the recovery period, monitor for dehydration and shock. Solid food should be taken only in extremely small amounts for the duration. Meat and plant broths will help the patient maintain his strength but be easy to digest. It is critical that the patient not be moved unless absolutely necessary in the early painful stages of this condition.

Part 5 Diarrhea. Diarrhea in the wilderness can not only be inconvenient and uncomfortable but can bring on a serious case of dehydration. There are two excellent treatments available to you in the wilderness. A strong tea made from the leaves of either Hudson Bay tea (also called Labrador tea) or lingonberry (see plant chapter) will help. The Hudson Bay tea is usually more effective but either will work, and both may be found under the snow in winter as well as growing fresh in the summer. When afflicted with diarrhea, you should take in a lot of liquids to replace the fluid you are losing and keep yourself well nourished. However, it would be better to be drinking broth than eating too much solid food until the condition clears up. Any of the sorrels or docks or other plants that are high in oxalic acid (such as rhubarb) will also be beneficial in controlling diarrhea.

Part 6 Barbed Hook. If you are not careful, it is easy to get a fish hook imbedded in a finger or other part of your body. If this happens, do not try to pull the hook out. It has a barb on it that will tear subcutaneous tissue and even tendons and ligaments. The hook must be pushed on through until the barb comes back out through the skin again (see figure # M-45) Then the barb must be either flattened or removed (see figure # M-46). Then you can safely pull the hook out. The area should then be disinfected and treated as a puncture wound.

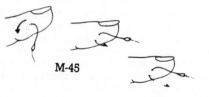

M-45

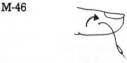

M-46

Section # 3—Suturing

In the wound section we referred to wound closure. Simple closure with butterfly bandages and steri-strips were shown. Both these work very well on smaller wounds that are on a part of the body not subjected to a lot of movement or stress. Steri-strips are preferred to close minor wounds on the face where it highly desirable to avoid scar formation. However, many wounds are too deep, too extensive or located in an area that must be functioning during the healing process and butterflies or steri-strips would simply not hold the wound closed. To have to close a wound a second time brings much greater risk of infection, scar formation and other complications. So, for larger wounds, you must suture.

When a wound is closed by any method, there must be no pockets of blood, air or foreign material left beneath the skin (see figure # M-47). These pockets will almost guarantee infection. Proper suturing technique will eliminate this problem. Stitching is no mystery and anyone can perform the procedure. You will need at least one needle holder (forceps with a needle groove) and the proper suture material. I believe that any good hand seamstress like most of our grandmother, could do a neater job than myself or any doctor. Suturing is simply sewing and the more you sew the better you get. It would be wise for everyone to pratice on two pieces of leather or a frying chicken before you cook it, until you get a good technique down.

Suture material is broken into two basic categories: Nondissolvable that will be used only on the surface where it can be removed once the wound has healed back together, and dissolvable that will be used when you must make stitches inside where they will not be accessible for removal, such as in a very deep wound where you must sew inner tissue and then close the outer tissue. The preferred non-dissolvable suture is monofilament. Braided silk is available but the texture of it allows greater chance of infection being introduced through the suture.

M-47

← WRONG!

pocket of blood

M-48

M-49

← RIGHT

WRONG

The most common suturing technique is shown in figure # M-48. Each stitch is tied separately from the rest. This is the easiest way to keep the edges of the wound lined up properly without puckering or mis-alignment, both of which retard healing and make for much greater scar formation. Each stitch should go to the bottom of the wound to prevent pockets and take in equal amount of tissue on both sides of the wound so that the edges will match up (see figure # M-49). Most stitches will be approximately ¼ inch apart. When suturing the face or hands you will want to use a finer suture material and the stitches will be approximately 1/8 inch apart. Here again, if possible use steri-strips on the face, but if you must suture, use a fine diameter like 6-0 monofilament. Sterile sutures come in a foil packet with needle already attached. For large wounds where considerable stress may be put on the sutures as the wound heals, like on the arm or leg, use a large suture like 3-0 monofilament. For most other suturing use 4-0 or 5-0 monofilament.

If you must do internal sutures, as with a very deep wound involving numerous layers of tissue, use 3-0 chromic gut. It will dissolve in time and will not cause a rejection response. Use the gut only on the internal layers. Then when you sew the skin use monofilament. Do not use the gut where it will be exposed to outside contaminants if possible (see figure # M-50).

Sutures should be tied off securely with a square knot (see figure # M-51). Make sure this knot is good and secure. Suturing can in most cases be accomplished without anesthetic if necessary but will range from moderately to extremely painful depending on the part of the body being sutured. If possible use xylocaine. It is a prescription drug, as is the syringe and nee-

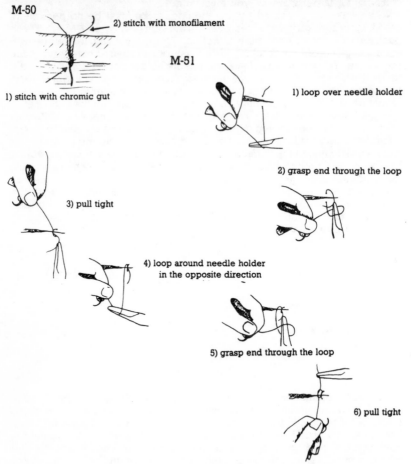

M-50

2) stitch with monofilament

1) stitch with chromic gut

M-51

1) loop over needle holder

2) grasp end through the loop

3) pull tight

4) loop around needle holder in the opposite direction

5) grasp end through the loop

6) pull tight

dle with which to inject it. It should be injected a little at a time just under the skin on the edge of the wound until the area is numb. You will need a doctor to prescribe these items for your kit.

Remember when suturing a wound to follow sanitary procedures rigorously. Leave sutures in for 10 days and then remove by carefully cutting with fine scissors (those found on a Swiss army knife work well for this). Grasp the knot with forceps, tweezers or your fingers and pull stitch out with a gentle, steady but firm pull (see figure # M-52).

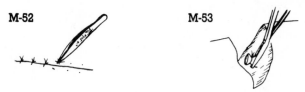

M-52 M-53

If you have a severed artery or vein that cannot be sealed off by direct pressure (as described in the section on controlling bleeding), you may have to tie it off with suture material. If available, clamp the blood vessel off with a hemostat (locking forceps that should be in your kit) upstream from the end and tie the blood vessel with a square knot (see figure # M-53). Irrigate, disinfect carefully and close the wound. Use chromic gut on the blood vessel as it will be internal.

CONCLUSION

As I write these final words, I am witnessing one of the most beautiful sunrises I have ever seen. I also see a fat snowshoe hare eyeing our garden. We don't mind, though. This year we planted enough for her too. She's a friend and also has a family to feed. It's the way of the wilderness and it's good.

The wilderness to me is life. It's a beautiful, rewarding and peaceful way of living. It's a place where a man can still enjoy freedom and communion with the real things around him. It's a place where a man can have the time to enjoy the beauty of a sunrise, the majesty of the endless mountains and the sound of silence where a man is still allowed the think, dream and pray in peace. Just to have the opportunity to hear the spruce trees speak in the wind and hear the bald eagle's unmistakable call is worth more than all the gold this world has. The eagle, the wolf and the bear have taught me what I know and the years of peace have given me the patience to listen and learn. The lessons can't be learned in a day, a month or a year. But if you find yourself in the wilderness, enjoy it and let it be your teacher. Nature can teach more in a single sunset than I can with this entire book.

This book is intended to give you a few ideas, facts and useful principles that may or may not apply to a given wilderness survival situation. Your own instincts, common sense and spirit are your most valuable assets and tools. No book can ever teach these and never allow the words of a book to take their place. I hope somehow, somewhere what I have written will help save a life that may have been lost to fear or lack of knowledge. Good-by my friend—maybe we'll pass each other on LIFE's trail someday.

REFERENCE APPENDIX
BEARS AND GUNS

The two most common questions I am asked are about the charges of bears and what is the best weapon for bear protection. As I mentioned before, bears are big, fast, strong and unpredictable. In most cases, a bear in the wild is not out to attack you. They can at times become real pests. They seem to enjoy tearing apart unattended cabins and equipment. If you leave your food or equipment where a bear can get at it, it's usually your fault. If you get in a bear's way and expect him to move over, in my estimation, you are a fool.

If you are in bear country and see signs of bear, making noise will almost always warn the bears and they will usually try to avoid you. If you are being quiet and you sneak up on a grizzly, you may have trouble. Bears do not like surprises. If you do come face-to-face with a bear, keep eye contact and slowly back off and get out of his area. Chances are good he will let you leave. If you come across a cute little bear cub, immediately put as much distance between it and yourself as you can. The mother will be close by and she will be very protective of her young. In this case she may kill you to make sure her cub is not harmed.

If a bear is eating the food you carelessly left in a bad spot, let him have it, unless you are capable of killing him. Try to avoid walking in dense brush, especially along salmon streams. If you have to walk in such areas, make noise and watch carefully. Try to walk the high ground where you can see all around you, and try to see a bear before it meets you. Figure where the bear is going and avoid getting in its way. These rules will keep you out of trouble with bears in most cases. If, however, you have the misfortune to get in a situation where a bear is attacking you, your best defense is to play dead. Remember you cannot out-fight him; you cannot out-run him and running away from any predator triggers a chase instinct. By playing dead, you may still be mauled but you will probably live. Trying to fight a bear is like attacking a tank with a golf club. There is an old story about hitting a bear on the nose but a bear can strike with a front paw far faster than you, and you will only further aggravate the bear if you try.

I do not advocate the needless killing of bears but because of their unpredictability, it is wise to carry an adequate firearm with you when in bear country. By adequate I don't mean a .38 special or a .357 magnum. These and similar handguns are designed to kill people, not bears and will not protect you from a grizzly. The only thing these guns can do for you in bear country is give you a false sense of security and get you into big trouble. When choosing a gun for self-defense against a bear, hand guns should be ruled out. Even the deadly .44 magnum will probably not do the job. I teach handgun safety and shooting and I usually can hit exactly what I'm shooting at but I wouldn't think of taking on a grizzly even with my .44 magnum.

Now that we've ruled out handguns, let me explain why. If we have a 700 pound grizzly mad and charging, a well-placed bullet will eventually kill the animal. The problem is that the animal has a lot of adrenalin worked up, weighs 700 pounds and is charging at an astonishing rate of speed. Even though the animal is virtually dead, he doesn't know it and he'll get you before he goes down from a mortal wound. What you must do to stop a charge is break major bones so the bear cannot mechanically function and collapses before he can reach you. A hand gun will not do this.

When hunting I use a .300 Weatherby magnum rifle. It has a very flat trajectory at long ranges and hits like a hand grenade. I don't believe there is an animal I can't kill with one shot at ranges up to 400 yards with this rifle.

But for a charging grizzly at close range, a 12 gauge shotgun loaded with rifled slugs is by far the finest bear-stopper I've seen. If you are not hunting but want a good bear defense gun, the 12 gauge with slugs is the answer. Then only remains that you learn to shoot it and shoot it accurately.

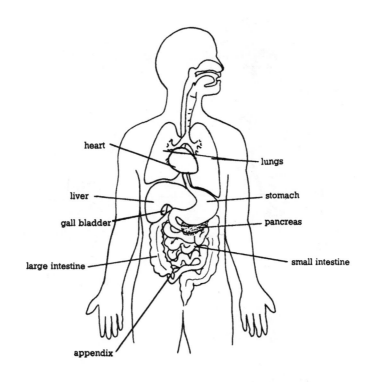

heart

lungs

liver

stomach

gall bladder

pancreas

large intestine

small intestine

appendix

major trunk organs

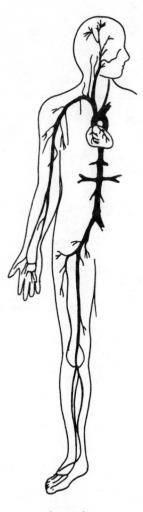

major arteries

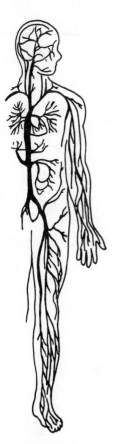

major veins

168

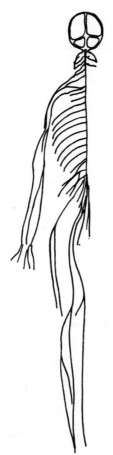

major nerves

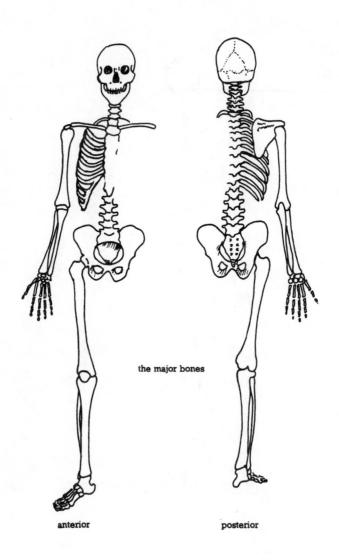

the major bones

anterior   posterior

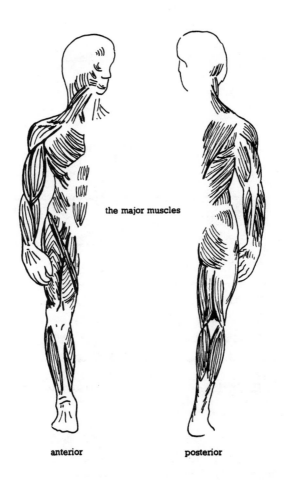

the major muscles

anterior   posterior

WIND CHILL CHART
WHAT THE THERMOMETER ACTUALLY READS

WIND SPEED (MPH) ↓	50	40	30	20	10	0	-10	-20	-30	-40	-50	-60
	WHAT IT EQUALS IN ITS EFFECT ON EXPOSED FLESH											
CALM	50	40	30	20	10	0	-10	-20	-30	-40	-50	-60
5	48	37	28	16	6	-5	-15	-26	-36	-47	-57	-68
10	40	28	16	4	-9	-21	-33	-46	-58	-70	-83	-95
15	36	22	9	-5	-18	-36	-45	-58	-72	-85	-99	-102
20	32	18	4	-10	-25	-39	-53	-67	-82	-96	-110	-124
25	30	16	0	-15	-29	-44	-59	-74	-83	-104	-113	-133
30	28	13	-2	-18	-33	-48	-63	-79	-94	-109	-125	-140
35	27	11	-4	-20	-35	-49	-64	-82	-98	-113	-129	-145
40	26	10	-6	-21	-37	-53	-69	-85	-102	-116	-132	-148

DANGER (center region)
GREAT DANGER (right region)

|← LITTLE DANGER IF PROPERLY CLOTHED →|← DANGER OF FREEZING EXPOSED FLESH →|

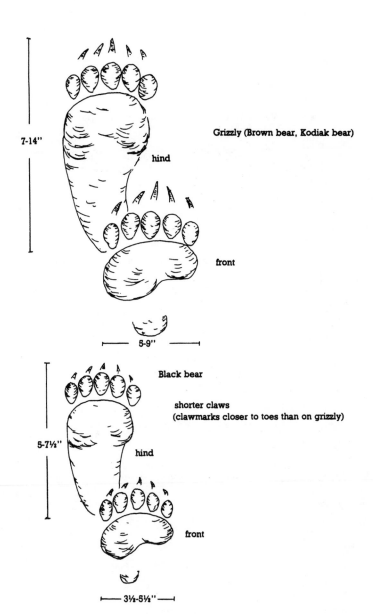

7-14"

Grizzly (Brown bear, Kodiak bear)

hind

front

5-9"

Black bear

shorter claws
(clawmarks closer to toes than on grizzly)

5-7½"

hind

front

3½-5½"

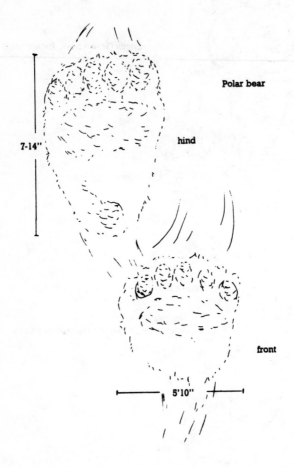

Polar bear

hind

7-14"

front

5'10"

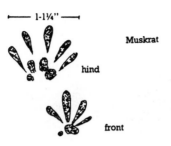

1-1¼"

Muskrat

hind

front

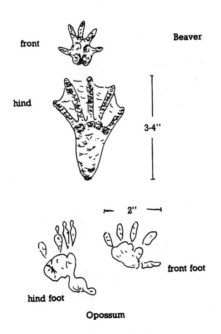

front

Beaver

hind

3-4"

2"

front foot

hind foot

Opossum

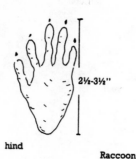

2½-3½"

hind   Raccoon

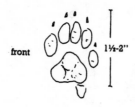

front   1½-2"

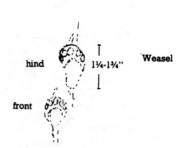

hind   1¼-1¾"   Weasel

front

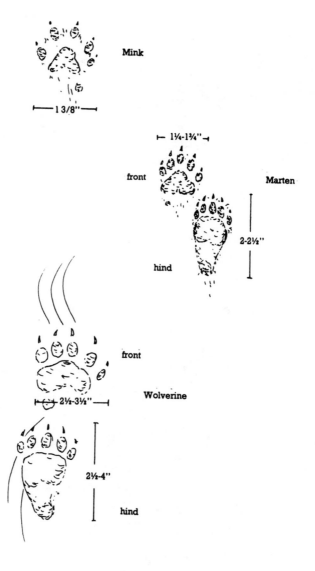

Mink

1 3/8"

1¼-1¾"

front

Marten

hind

2-2½"

front

Wolverine

2½-3½"

2½-4"

hind

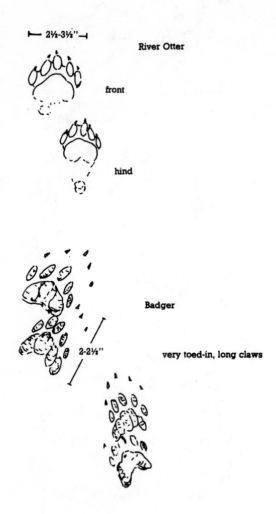

├─ 2½-3½" ─┤

River Otter

front

hind

Badger

2-2½"

very toed-in, long claws

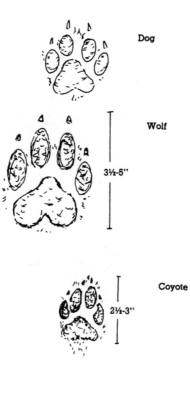

Dog

Wolf

3½-5''

Coyote

2½-3''

Red Fox

2-2½''

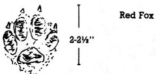

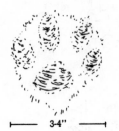

Lynx

├─── 3-4" ───┤

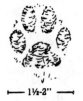

Bobcat

├─ 1½-2" ─┤

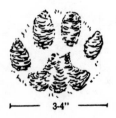

Cougar

├─── 3-4" ───┤

180

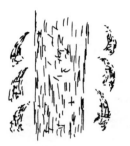 Seal

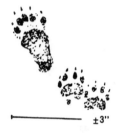 Squirrel

±1"

±3"

front 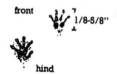 1/8-5/8"

Voles & Mice

hind

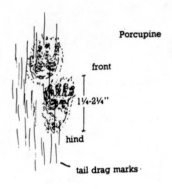

Porcupine

front

1¼-2¼"

hind

— tail drag marks

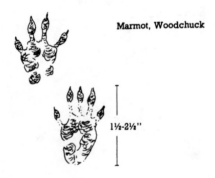

Marmot, Woodchuck

1½-2½"

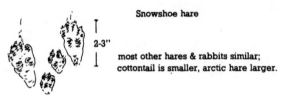

Snowshoe hare

2-3"

most other hares & rabbits similar;
cottontail is smaller, arctic hare larger.

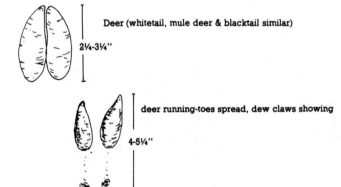

Deer (whitetail, mule deer & blacktail similar)

2¼-3¼"

deer running-toes spread, dew claws showing

4-5¼"

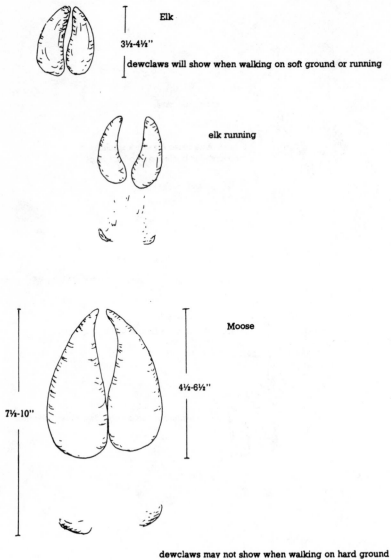

Elk

3½-4½"

dewclaws will show when walking on soft ground or running

elk running

Moose

4½-6½"

7½-10"

dewclaws may not show when walking on hard ground

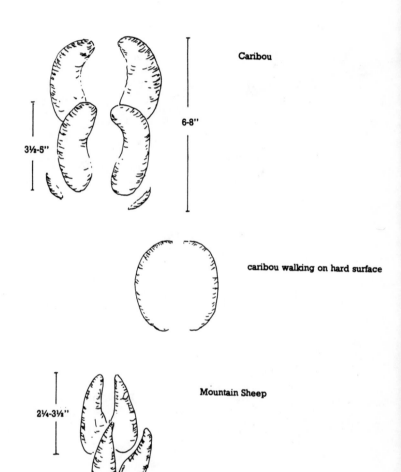

Caribou

6-8"

3½-5"

caribou walking on hard surface

Mountain Sheep

2¼-3½"

185

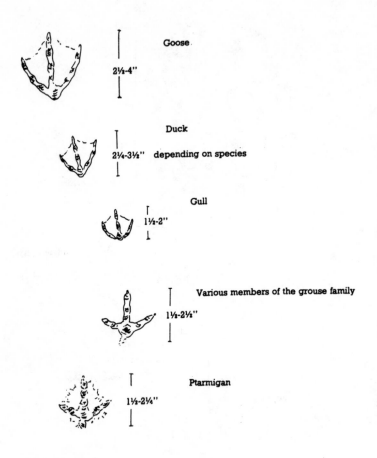

Goose

2½-4″

Duck

2¼-3½″   depending on species

Gull

1½-2″

Various members of the grouse family

1½-2½″

Ptarmigan

1½-2¼″

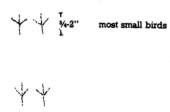 ¾-2" most small birds

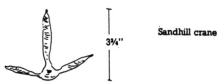

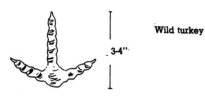 3¾" Sandhill crane

Wild turkey

3-4"

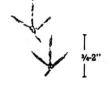 ¾-2" most shore birds

├── 1-5" ──┤

various species of frog

├── 1½-12" ──┤

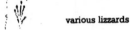

various lizzards

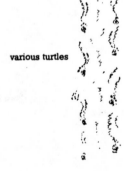

various turtles

Universal Air-to Ground Signals

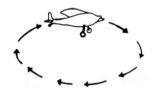

message received but not understood

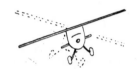

message received & understood

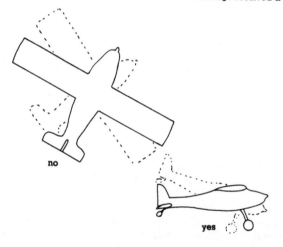

no

yes

Universal Body Signals

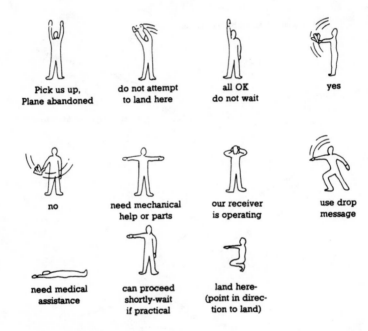

Pick us up,
Plane abandoned

do not attempt
to land here

all OK
do not wait

yes

no

need mechanical
help or parts

our receiver
is operating

use drop
message

need medical
assistance

can proceed
shortly-wait
if practical

land here-
(point in direc-
tion to land)

NOTE: To assist the rescue plane landing on snow or ice, place green boughs or some readily recognizable objects along landing strip to give the pilot some depth perception.

Universal Ground-to Air Emergency Signals

I
serious injuries-
require doctor

II
require medical
supplies

X
unable to
proceed

F
require food &
water

require firearms
& ammunition

K
indicate
direction to
proceed

↑
am proceeding
in this direction

will attempt
to take off

aircraft badly
damaged

△
probably safe to
land here

LL
all well

L
require fuel
& oil

N
NO

Y
YES

⌐L
not
understood

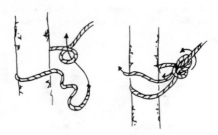

Bowline-strong, will not slip

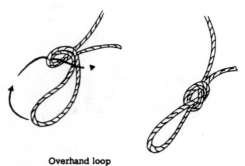

Overhand loop

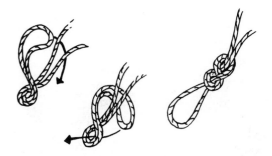

Figure 8- easier to untie than the overhand loop

Water knot- to join two ropes

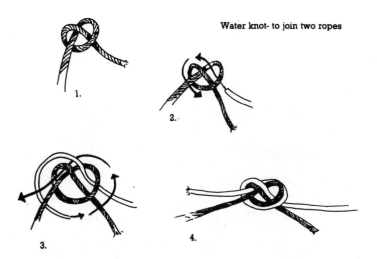

1.

2.

3.

4.

193

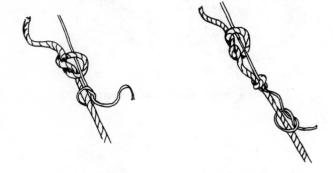

Fisherman's knot- for joining 2 ropes of different sizes

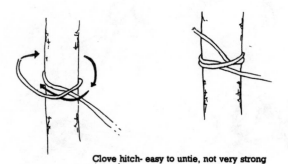

Clove hitch- easy to untie, not very strong

194

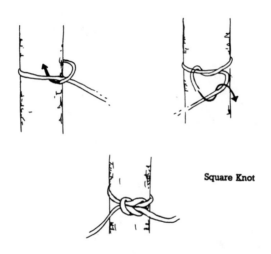

Square Knot